FERTILITY
MINDSET & MELTDOWNS

Cherish
EDITIONS

READER REVIEWS

Serena G., UK
"I would recommend this book to anyone struggling with their fertility."

Louise F., Canada
"How I wish I'd had this book on my fertility journey!"

Stef M., UK
"Lisa's insights helped me to calm my mind and reframe the whole fertility process."

Rebecca W., UK
"This book is the perfect guide for what can be a terrifying, tough and lonely time."

ABOUT THE AUTHOR

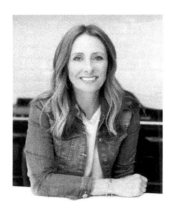

Lisa Ashworth is a writer and qualified coach who endured a ten-year struggle to conceive a baby with many personal and medical challenges along the way. She has written about the huge toll this took on her mental health and is passionate about sharing how she transformed her fertility plan by learning to manage her mindset. Lisa finally gave birth to triplets at the age of 41 and then worked as a fertility coach, supporting clients who were trying to conceive. She is now a career coach and writer, and she lives in the UK's Surrey Hills with her husband and their 11-year-old triplets.

FERTILITY
MINDSET & MELTDOWNS

How to take control of your emotions
while trying to conceive

Could your mindset be your missing link?

Lisa Ashworth

Cherish
EDITIONS

Published in 2023 by Cherish Editions
An imprint of Shaw Callaghan Ltd

UK Office
The Stanley Building
7 Pancras Square
Kings Cross
London N1C 4AG

US Office
On Point Executive Center, Inc
3030 N Rocky Point Drive W
Suite 150
Tampa, FL 33607
www.triggerhub.org

A CIP catalogue record for this book is available upon request
from the British Library
ISBN: 978-1-915680-65-5
Ebook ISBN: 978-1-915680-66-2

Cover design by More Visual Ltd.
Typeset by Lapiz Digital Services

For Jessica, Harry and Max... worth the wait.

FOREWORD

Many women dream of the time that they will become a mother. A large majority do not realize the heavy toll that the journey to motherhood will take on their emotional well-being. Lisa Ashworth provides practical tips and guidance to navigating your own mental health through fertility challenges. Her experience is rooted in her own first-hand highs and lows along this difficult path. She unravels the intricate connection between the internal mindset and the external physical states that are essential to a successful conception.

Dr Caitlin Scott
GP – Women's Health and Hormones
Guildford, UK

IS THIS BOOK FOR YOU?

This book is for anyone who is struggling with the mental strain of trying to get pregnant. It doesn't matter if you've been trying for three months or three years, if you're trying to get pregnant for the first time, or if you already have a child. You might be trying to conceive naturally or be heading down the IVF route, with either a diagnosed medical condition or no obvious explanation as to why you can't get pregnant. You could be female or male, in a heterosexual relationship or a same-sex partnership. Everyone's story is different, but the common thread is how mentally tough the journey is.

This book is for you if you feel that your emotions are out of control and trying to conceive is taking over your life. Perhaps you feel like a cloud of depression is hanging over you, or that you go through your days with an underlying sadness about your situation. You could be anxious about whether or not you'll get pregnant and feel helpless about what to do next. You may feel angry that everyone else seems to be pregnant and you're not, or perhaps you are isolated and unable to talk to anyone about it.

This book is for you if the whole situation is getting you down and you've run out of ideas of where to go next. I can't control what's going on in your head and I certainly can't get you pregnant, but what I can do is tell you how I discovered that managing my mindset was the missing link in my quest to get pregnant. I can share with you the simple tools and exercises that I learned which will help you take control of your thoughts and make them work for you, not against you.

This book also provides useful insights and tips for managing some of the toughest aspects of your fertility journey. My Survival Guides, at the end of the book, feature a range of 14 different scenarios that you may encounter, including how to handle intrusive questions, how to survive a baby shower and how to juggle fertility treatment with work.

What this book won't do is give you lots of medical advice or diagnose specific fertility problems you might have. I'm not a doctor or qualified psychologist. But I am someone who has been on the exact same journey and was for ten years.

I know exactly the pain and agony you are going through and all the different situations that can trigger what I call a "mindset meltdown". I had tried everything to get pregnant – and I literally mean everything! I know how desperate you can become when you want a baby so badly, and how you will try anything if you think it will deliver you that positive test. From medical drugs and fertility treatments, through to alternative therapies and holistic medicine – I have tried some crazy things and spent an absolute fortune too!

With this book, I hope you will reach a place where you are facing this journey with renewed energy and positivity, whatever stage you are at and however long you have been trying. There is so much written about the mind-body connection to help with all aspects of life, but this book focuses it all on fertility. You may be thinking, "Can it really be that simple?" or "That will never work for me", but if you feel the same way I did, and you have no idea where to turn to next, it could be exactly what you need. You don't need much to get going – just an open mind, daily commitment and practice. Surely a baby is worth it.

CONTENTS

PART ONE

INTRODUCTION

DESPERATE TO CONCEIVE

It was yet another family event, a christening this time. I stood next to my friends, all dressed up, and cooed at the baby with a smile plastered on my face. I watched the other children running around happily as I listened to the parents, sharing tales of their latest proud moments. I had become an expert at wearing the mask by then, pretending everything was fine and making small talk about nothing at all.

To any onlooker, my life sounded fantastic. I chatted happily about how well my job was going, how I'd signed up for a running challenge, how we were planning another holiday. Life was pretty good, so what did I have to complain about? I had the husband, the career and all the time in the world to enjoy life to the full.

But I could feel the elephant in the room. No one dared ask how "it" was going. They all knew it had been going on for far too long. They were desperately sympathetic and yet terrified of saying the wrong thing. Instead, they made light of it all. They joked about how tired they were as parents, how they would love to have time to go for run and how a holiday without kids would be heavenly. They thought they were making me feel better, but to me, it felt as though they were rubbing my nose in it even more.

I was the one who wanted the sleepless nights and the family holidays. I was dreaming about staying in my PJs all day and pushing a buggy around. I was even excited about changing nappies and getting up in the middle of the night! Rose-tinted glasses, I know, but I knew I was missing out. I'd reached that time in my life where I'd had enough of thinking of myself and I was ready to be a mum. Sadly, it wasn't happening. Before I knew it, the weeks of trying turned into months, and over time the months became years.

As I gazed around the room at the seemingly perfect families in front of me, familiar feelings of envy and resentment bubbled up. It was time to leave. When I returned home that night, I curled up on the bathroom floor and sobbed. I was exhausted from wearing the mask all day, yet again, and pretending everything was fine. I was so desperately sad that I couldn't get pregnant, and the thought of facing life without being a mum was overwhelming. Time was ticking and nothing was changing. I felt totally out of control and anxious about the future, and I had no idea what to do next. More than anything, I felt alone. No one really understood what I was going through, and while all my friends were playing happy families, I was the one being left behind.

My fertility journey lasted ten years. They were long, desperate years full of emotional highs and lows, and numerous failed pregnancy tests. Trying to conceive became a hidden obsession of mine. Every month, I monitored my cycle religiously, over-analysing every little sign that I might be pregnant. I left no stone unturned in my quest to get pregnant. I took every fertility test under the sun, tried so many different drugs and, of course, every natural remedy out there – who knew the Internet would be a source of so many wacky fertility-boosting claims? Over the years, I tried more than a few. Finally, my husband and I turned to fertility treatment and spent thousands of pounds on IVF. It was all emotionally and mentally exhausting and a complete drain on our bank balance.

My story did end happily as you will read, but for a long time I felt as though I wouldn't get there. The mental challenge of trying to conceive was unlike anything I had ever experienced.

It was overwhelming and dominated my life for those ten years. I was so desperate to be pregnant that I lost sight of what was good in my life, and I came close to breaking point many times. It seemed like everyone around me was falling pregnant very easily, and I was always the one who couldn't get there. The monthly cycle was a familiar pattern filled with fresh hope at the start, leading to anxiety and then disappointment as my period arrived yet again.

One of the biggest frustrations was that it felt completely out of my control. I'm the first to admit I am a bit of a control freak – I've always been used to calling the shots and doing what I wanted when I wanted, but this fertility problem came along and stopped me in my tracks. It was the first time in my life that I wasn't in control, or so I thought. And, over time, that led to the most frustrating, depressing and lonely experience of my life.

When I look back on those ten years, I felt a bit like a swan. On the surface I appeared very calm and in control, gliding happily through my life, despite not being pregnant. But underneath, the mental challenge of the journey was a daily struggle, and I was paddling frantically to get through the days. No one had a clue what was really going on, as I covered it all up. I worked really hard to be positive every day, despite dealing with the fact that the one thing I desperately wanted – to be pregnant – wasn't happening.

Everything changed...

When I was sobbing on the bathroom floor that night, I had no idea that, in a matter of months, things would finally change and I would be pregnant – and not only with one baby. Incredibly, I fell pregnant with triplets at the age of 40. I couldn't have made it up. I went on to have the most fantastic pregnancy, with everything going smoothly, despite all the risks the consultants warned me about. The babies arrived at

35 weeks, and the most crazy but joyful new chapter in our lives began. But that's another story.

This is the story of how I got there. When I was almost at the point of giving up, I discovered what, for me, was the missing link. I have now learnt that there are parts of this journey that you can control, and they have a significant impact on what happens to you. I look back and see the mismatch between what was happening to me on the outside with all the practical, positive things I was doing to try to get pregnant, and all the negative thoughts and feelings that consumed me inside. They were total opposites.

Have you ever tried to go for a run when you feel exhausted? Eat a big dinner when you're not hungry? Or kick off a new project when your heart's not in it? It's not easy. In fact, it's almost impossible. I have learnt that what you think about has a huge impact on your life and will determine your behaviour, the actions you take and the experiences you attract. I was trying very hard to get pregnant on the outside, but inside I had totally lost faith. In this book, I will show you exactly how I learnt to take control of my mindset and make it work for me, not against me. Once I mastered some easy-to-learn tools, I got my fertility journey back on track, started enjoying my life again, and everything changed... very quickly. And not long afterwards, I finally achieved the result I had been waiting for.

CHAPTER 1

MY STORY – A MEDICAL AND EMOTIONAL ROLLERCOASTER

I want to start by telling you my story. When I was on this journey, other people's stories always inspired me and gave me hope. I would often look for tenuous links to my own situation, and I found it very reassuring to read that there were other people out there as desperate as I was, with similar challenges to me, who got there in the end.

I also appreciate that not everyone wants to read about happy endings. I went through a phase like that too, so I get it. Those happy endings can be cruel reminders of what you don't have now, and it hurts. They might also seem idealistic, ignoring the reality of what you're facing. If you feel this way, that's totally fine, just skip this chapter. You have to do what works for your own mindset. But remember, I was exactly where you are right now – I had a whole host of challenges facing me, and I did get there in the end.

For those who are looking for hope, my story may provide inspiration. Anything you can do to keep the faith and remind yourself that this can happen for you is a good thing. Hopefully, knowing that I became pregnant with triplets at the age of 40, after five failed IVFs and ten years of trying, will give you the determination to keep going.

I first started officially "trying" when I was 30 and in my first marriage. Nothing happened, but I wasn't too worried because I was still quite young and could reassure myself that it might take a few months to fall pregnant. As time went on, more of my friends were getting pregnant and having families, and I started to face the reality that it wasn't happening for me. Cue all the standard tests, which showed there was nothing medically wrong, so I dabbled in a few fertility drugs like Clomid and Metformin, and I tried a couple of IUIs, but still no baby.

On top of this, my marriage was breaking down. I got married relatively young at 26, but sadly it didn't work out. Don't get me wrong, he was a great guy, and we had a full life at the time with a brilliant circle of friends. On the outside you wouldn't have realized there was anything wrong. We were in our 20s, working hard, having fun and seeing the world by going on great holidays, but deep down I knew it wasn't right. We simply didn't enjoy the same things in life and, as time went on, we were drifting apart and doing less and less together. However, the one thing we did have in common was that we both wanted kids. Looking back now, the quest to become pregnant kept us together longer than we needed to be. We both secretly hoped that I would be pregnant each month and a new family life would bring us back together. But it wasn't to be. The baby never came, and instead my marriage became empty. By the time I was 35, I was desperately unhappy but worried I was too old to start again (looking back now, what was I thinking?!). After a lot of soul searching, I eventually found the courage to make a change. And isn't hindsight an amazing thing, because in many ways it was a relief for both of us that I didn't become pregnant back then.

It took me a while to recover, but then my life improved. In fact, the next couple of years were great. I bought my own place to live, my career was flying high, and I dated a bit to restore my faith in men. I generally regained my mojo, and it was fantastic to have no fertility pressures hanging over me. But I was keen to meet someone new. At the time I was working hard and all my friends were married, so I didn't really go anywhere to meet people. Therefore, I had no problem signing up to a dating site. I launched myself in with renewed enthusiasm and I have to say it was quite fun at first. Back then, it was still a relatively new way of meeting people, and fairly civilized – none of this swiping left and right!

But after a while I felt jaded from it all. Mr Right hadn't appeared, so I decided to take a break and cancel my membership. My account literally had two weeks before it expired, and it was in that fortnight that "Rob from Beaconsfield" popped up as a suggested match. He had just joined the site, and I was about to leave it. We had our first date and hit it off immediately. I know it sounds cheesy, but it was pretty much love at first sight. We just knew it was right, and when you know it's right, you want to get on with everything right there and then. We were engaged after three months, moved into together soon after and started trying to get pregnant that same year. We were both a few years away from 40 and we wanted children. So, with my previous difficulties at the back of my mind, we decided to start trying. I was intrigued to see whether the same thing would happen or if it would be different with someone new.

Despite my positive outlook, sadly there was no baby. I had thought it might be different this time, especially now I had found "the one" and felt like everything was meant to be. Cue more tests, investigations and the hugely frustrating diagnosis that there was nothing medically wrong with either of us, but I still wasn't getting pregnant.

Once again, I tried everything I could to increase my chances. I went on various fertility diets, took all the vitamins under the sun and tried numerous alternative therapies. Nothing made any difference and, as time went on, I fell deeper and deeper into despair.

We had our first IVF round and nothing happened. "It's okay," the consultant said, "it's very common not to work the first time." "Great!" I said. "Let's do another round then." We paid our second £4,000, which I think these days is quite a reasonable fee for a round of IVF, but was a lot to us back then. Thank goodness we had some spare cash from a redundancy settlement – that made it a lot easier. Incredibly, this time it was positive! We couldn't believe it! Crushingly, though, the joy was short-lived. I had a very early miscarriage, and at the six-week scan, there was nothing there to see.

But, ever the optimist, I was sure it would work next time as we had been so close before. So, off we went again into a new round of IVF, paying another £4,000 and having a load more scans and injections, not to mention juggling it all with two busy jobs. The third one didn't work either. We were devastated, and it took a while to get over that one. We decided to take a break and do something positive – we got married. We had a beautiful winter wedding and amazing honeymoon. When we got home, I was feeling super relaxed and blissfully happy with my new husband, and so I couldn't wait to start again with IVF number four. Surely this one would work. But it didn't. Despite everything going okay with the actual process, there was still no baby, and we were another £4,000 down.

This time I didn't bounce back. I was 39 and about to turn 40. I had four failed IVF attempts behind me, the money had run out, and my biological clock was ticking. 40 had always been a milestone for me. I wanted to be pregnant by the time I was 40 at the very latest. In my head my time was running out and I was a failure. My mind was consumed with worry and anxiety about what was going to happen. *Would I ever be pregnant? And why was this happening to me?*

I was losing faith and feeling totally overwhelmed by the situation. I was so low, and life felt hopeless. What more could I do? I thought I'd tried everything. I couldn't face my high-flying job anymore either, and juggling it with the invasive treatment had become really tough. I had a decision to make. Either I turned 40, put all this behind me and focused on enjoying a new life without our own children, or I packed in my job and tried to work out a last-ditch plan for my pregnancy quest.

As anyone who is on this journey knows, it is hugely difficult to draw a line under your pregnancy hopes and give up trying. So, after much debate, I left my job. We calculated that I could afford to take three months off, and during that time I would focus on rebuilding my strength – physically and mentally – and work out what the heck we were going to do next. On top of everything else, we hadn't long moved into our house, so the renovation project would be a distraction too.

It was so nice to be at home. I hadn't realized how exhausted I was, both mentally and physically, and a break from corporate life after 20 years was just the tonic I needed. It was during those few months that I did a lot of reading. I've always been into self-help tools, and I was trying to find a new spark of inspiration that would help dig me out of my hole. I knew something had to change but I didn't know what.

I started reading more and more about mindset. I knew there was a lot going on for me mentally on this journey, and a host of emotions were constantly swirling round my head, but until that point I didn't really appreciate the effect this was having on my mindset and how I was feeling day to day. I certainly didn't realize I could control any of it. However, the more I read, the more I realized there was a complete mismatch between all the negative thoughts and feelings I was having deep down inside, and everything positive I was doing on a practical and physical level to become pregnant. This mismatch was creating a major conflict internally, and that was contributing to my negative results.

There was so much out there on this topic. So many different people were fundamentally saying the same thing – that what you think about comes about, and if you change your mindset, you can change your life. Was it really that easy? I have to say I was sceptical at first. I thought I had always been a positive person, and having a baby was something I really wanted, after all! Why on earth would I be negative about it?! But as I read on, I could see that although I thought I was being positive, a lot of my inner thinking had become so negative and automatic that I couldn't control it happening. Those negative thoughts led to negative feelings, which had a massive impact on my actions and behaviour day to day.

I realized that although I tried to shut these thoughts out, hide them from the world and pretend like everything was fine, they were subconsciously dominating my thinking every day and, therefore, creating similar results in my life. It was a light-bulb moment for me. I learned that the brain is like a muscle, and you can train it to work for you or against you. When it works against you, negative thinking can become such a reflex that you may not even notice how critical you're being of yourself, and that has a knock-on effect on your behaviour and the results you see in your life. When it works for you, and you start to control the thoughts in your head, you can ultimately change your life for the better.

There was so much written on this topic and so many tools and techniques out there, but eventually, with a bit of trial and error, I developed a handful that worked for me and began using them daily. I was training my brain, like completing a daily workout at the gym. It was simple, but it wasn't always easy – breaking the habits of a lifetime never is. But consistency proved to be the key, and very soon things started changing. I felt the joy creep back into my life and I became a glass-half-full person again. I noticed things going right instead of wrong, and I definitely regained my energy and confidence. I was delighted and, slowly, life started to feel okay again.

At this point I wasn't considering another IVF round. I had convinced myself that doing the same thing over and over again and expecting a different result was surely the definition of madness. But my husband wouldn't let it go, and I found myself becoming open to it again and seeing the process in a new, more positive light. Then, my mother-in-law rang one day and offered to pay for a round for us. Another positive step. Everything seemed to be falling into place, so I felt that trying IVF again was the right thing to do. I agreed to give it another go, but we decided it would be our absolute last one.

This time it felt different. Something had definitely shifted inside me. I was continuing to practise the tools I had learnt and I had a new energy about me. This time I found myself booking an appointment with the consultant and pushing for things to be done differently. I explained that there was no way I was doing IVF again without something changing. Surely there were more tests they could do, or different techniques they could try? It turned out there were more tests, which were normally only performed after you'd had three miscarriages. I'd only had one miscarriage, so these tests had never been offered to me before. We paid privately for the tests, and they highlighted one possible factor. It was a very minor issue, and the consultant said there was a chance it could be impacting my pregnancy success, but that it also may not be relevant at all. It was a long shot. But with my persistence, he agreed to tweak the drugs and do things slightly differently, just in case.

The next IVF cycle was pretty similar to before. I'd never been one of those women who produced loads of eggs, and this time they removed five eggs ready to fertilize, which was pretty average for me. But I still felt much more positive. It was at this point that they sat us down for a frank discussion. They knew it was our last round of IVF and I was now 40 years old, so they were trying to persuade us to put three embryos back in to increase our chances. We were totally gobsmacked! On the one hand, it hadn't worked so far, so what were the chances of all three embryos taking? But on the other hand – three babies? Who on earth could cope with that? We were told it was very unlikely that all three would take and that we had until the next morning to make our decision. A lot of soul searching went on that night, I can tell you. But in the end, because it was our last round, we decided to go for it. Were we totally bonkers? I have no idea, but it felt right. Whatever happened, we would know in our heart of hearts that we had tried absolutely everything.

However, fate always has a hand in things, and in the morning, we were told that only two embryos were good enough to put back. My heart sank. I couldn't help but wonder if those two embryos would be any good since the other three weren't. Maybe they were the best of a bad bunch? But

I pushed that thought out of my mind and kept using all the tools I had learnt, and we started our two-week wait with a positive outlook.

We survived the agonizing two-week wait as normal, despite me falling down the stairs on day ten, which was definitely a test of my mindset! Eventually, the day came for the pregnancy test. It was first thing in the morning on Bonfire Night, and we were both lying in bed. I couldn't bear to look at it. I passed it straight to Rob, who stared at it for what seemed to me like an eternity. Eventually, he turned to me blankly and said, "Pregnant." I couldn't believe it and grabbed the test to see for myself. Well, there it was: a big, fat, positive result at the age of 40 after five IVF rounds.

Two weeks later we were sitting at the ultrasound, waiting to see if we were still pregnant and what was going on inside. Quite quickly the sonographer announced excitedly that it was twins and that she could see two sacs! Wow... we were overjoyed! We finally had a proper pregnancy that we could see on the screen. We could see the tiny heartbeats, it was incredible! All the way through this process, we had secretly hoped for twins, and after such a long wait, we were overwhelmed to realize we would have our ready-made family after all. This was the best news ever, and we could hardly believe it. But while we were hugging each other with tears of joy and relief in our eyes, we noticed that the sonographer was completely silent, staring intently at the screen. I nudged Rob and nodding toward her, asked if everything was okay. "Err yes," she said. "Everything is great, it's just that I think there are actually three babies in there!"

What?! Three babies?! Where had they come from? And how? The next ten minutes were a complete blur while we tried to get our heads around what had happened. Not only was the pregnancy successful, but one of the embryos had randomly split into two, giving us identical twins, plus one more. It was unbelievable! We'd had four failed attempts with so many years of disappointments. Against all the odds, and at the age of 40, not only did the final one work, but we ended up with three babies.

To say we were in shock was an understatement, and that shock continued throughout the pregnancy, right up until our two boys and our little girl arrived safely at 35 weeks.

What worked for me...

This book is about what worked for me in the end. At my lowest point, I discovered the tools that changed everything for me mentally. They were simple tools that you can use too. I was at rock bottom, highly anxious and feeling totally out of control. I had no idea why I wasn't becoming pregnant, and I had run out of ideas of where to go next. My mind was automatically thinking the worst, often without me realizing it. My internal chatter was highly critical, and I was talking to myself in a way I wouldn't talk to my worst enemy! All this was in complete contrast to the positive things I was doing on the outside to try and get pregnant. No wonder nothing was happening.

This mindset meltdown had caused me to become completely closed off to new ideas, ignoring opportunities around me that might move me closer to my goal of being pregnant. Once I discovered these tools and used them daily, I slowly started to regain control of the thoughts in my head. I noticed that I enjoyed my life again and I retrained my brain to appreciate what was already good around me. I started to behave differently, developing a new positive energy toward my fertility journey. I had sprung into action and I was open to new ideas. I had no hesitation in exploring the opportunities around me and I had a new belief and faith that everything would be okay.

You too can use these tools to retrain your thoughts and keep your mindset on track. With these methods, you can get back to feeling positive and in control, and you can find that boost of energy you need to move your journey forward. And, hopefully, you will be a lot happier along the way.

PART TWO

THE FERTILITY MINDSET MELTDOWN

Before we dive into the tools, it's important for you to work out exactly where you need help. Everyone is different and, as you go through this fertility journey, you will have your own situations that trigger you. When I was on my journey, I felt like I had a publicly happy life on the outside and a hidden struggle going on inside. I developed secret rituals and obsessions that showed up on a daily basis. They were slightly alarming things I found myself doing, often without realizing, and I felt so ashamed at first that I wouldn't even tell my husband about them. I was worried he wouldn't understand and might even think I had lost the plot! I thought, *Surely no one else would lower themselves to this desperate behaviour*? You're probably wondering what things I was doing. Well, I've gone public with my list now, and you can find it in this section. Hiding these obsessions only added to my feelings of loneliness, causing me to withdraw even more.

In this section you will also read about the traits of what I call a *Fertility Mindset Meltdown*. This meltdown in your head can happen to even the most positive of people – I should know, I was one of them. I went from being a positive, can-do, go-getter to becoming obsessed, anxious and hugely negative about my ability to get pregnant. But none of this played out publicly. On the outside, I carried on as normal and said I was fine if anyone asked. I did all the things I should have been doing to get pregnant. The negative stuff was what was going on in my head, and often I didn't even realize it was happening or the effect it was having on me. If you have secretly felt this way on your own journey, I want to reassure you that you are not alone. You are not the only one thinking or doing slightly crazy things, and I'm pleased to say there is a way to change things. So, let's talk a bit more about what's going on mentally when you find yourself having a mindset meltdown.

CHAPTER 2

EMOTIONAL AND EASILY TRIGGERED

People experience disappointments in life all the time. It could be a job-interview rejection, a relationship break-up or a house sale falling through, to name a few. These are all huge, important events. It's awful when they go wrong, and it's only natural that you will feel disappointed. But somehow the disappointment of not falling pregnant seems immense compared to other events in life. Getting pregnant is quite simply a life goal. Reproduction is what we were put on this earth to do, and it can be easy to take it for granted that you will become pregnant when the time is right for you. When you've decided you want a baby and it doesn't happen, it can be devastating. Multiply that disappointment by days, months and years, and that is bound to take its toll on you emotionally.

It doesn't matter what stage of the journey you're at, trying for a baby is definitely an emotional process. You might still be trying naturally each month, or be much further down the line with some form of fertility treatment. You could be trying for your first baby, or this could be your second or third child. Whatever stage you're at, the cycle of emotions you experience each month will be a rollercoaster. And everyone is different. I have always been a bit of a control freak, so at the start of the journey, I felt irritated and annoyed that I wasn't getting what I wanted. As time went on, and after many years of trying, that turned into a constant state of anxiety and a daily sadness that I carried around inside of me.

As you will learn in this book, the way you think and feel affects the way you behave, so not only do you feel emotionally low on this journey, but your life can start to crumble a bit too. You might start to feel as if your life is on pause, or be too overwhelmed to take any action to move forward with your medical journey. You might see cracks in your relationship, or isolate yourself from social events, particularly if they involve children.

Exercise: Your top five emotions

Let's start by identifying how your own fertility journey is affecting you emotionally.

When you're trying to conceive, the emotions you are likely to experience will vary hugely and can be different for everyone. But when I started helping women going through this journey, I noticed many common themes.

Have a look at the list of emotions below and consider how they apply to your own fertility journey. How do you feel right now? How have you felt at your toughest times? And which of these emotions resonate with your situation the most?

- **Anxiety** – I am anxious about the future; I worry about not getting pregnant; I feel anxious about what could be wrong with me; I worry that a fertility treatment won't work.
- **Sadness** – I am sad that I'm not pregnant, that I can't have the family I want.
- **Grief** – I feel a sense of loss for the baby I want but can't have; I feel grief for not being able to become a mother.
- **Inadequacy** – Why me? How come everyone else gets pregnant easily? I'm not good enough – this is all I deserve.
- **Depression** – I feel overwhelmed by my situation; I'm struggling to cope with everything; I find it hard to get through life day to day.

- **Paranoia** – There must be something wrong with me; everyone is talking about me; everyone feels sorry for me; I see pregnant women wherever I go.
- **Sensitivity** – I take things personally; I am easily upset or offended; I feel awkward talking about my fertility journey.
- **Emotional** – I cry easily; I have regular emotional outbursts; I am very easily triggered; I bottle up my emotions.
- **Anger** – I feel bitter or resentful that this isn't happening for me; I am frustrated that I'm not pregnant; I feel angry at everyone else for having children.
- **Envy** – I feel jealous of anyone who is pregnant; I am envious of families I see out and about; I am jealous of friends who are pregnant.
- **Bitterness** – It's not fair that she got pregnant straight away; I can't stand to be around them as they're pregnant.
- **Loneliness** – I am the only one who isn't pregnant; I can't talk to anyone about this – no one understands what I'm going through.
- **Disappointment** – Another month without a baby; my treatment didn't work; I'm not pregnant again.
- **Frustration** – Despite everything I'm doing, I'm still not pregnant; time is running out for me; why isn't it working?
- **Out of control** – I've tried everything but I'm still not pregnant; there is nothing wrong with me, but I still can't get pregnant; I have no idea what to do next.
- **Obsession** – I can't stop thinking about getting pregnant; everywhere I go I see pregnant women; I'm constantly wondering if I'm pregnant this month – I can't plan anything in case I'm pregnant, I can't eat that in case I'm pregnant.
- **Over-analytical** – What's that twinge? Are my boobs bigger? Is that blood? I need to look that up on Google!
- **Negativity** – This will never happen to me; I'm not going to get pregnant; I'm always the one this doesn't happen to; that treatment won't work for me.

- **Low energy** – I can't face life today; I have no energy to move forward; I make lots of excuses not to take action; I am drifting through my fertility journey.

Consider these emotions and identify the top five that affect you the most.

Make a note of these below and be specific in describing what each one means to you.

You will need these for later in the book when you create your mindset action plan.

MY TOP FIVE EMOTIONS

1.

2.

3.

4.

5.

Exercise: Find your triggers

It's also important to think about your emotional triggers. What type of events trigger a mindset meltdown for you? These could be situations you are confronted with day to day or something more ad-hoc. It could be a big, obvious trigger, like your best friend getting pregnant or your period arriving at the end of the month. Or, it could be something seemingly minor, like seeing a pregnancy reference on TV that has a huge impact on how you feel. Look at the list below – which are your biggest triggers?

- Comparison to others, especially happy families
- Monthly period arriving
- Social events with families
- Friends being pregnant
- Lack of understanding from your partner
- Baby showers
- People asking how you are
- Hospital appointments
- Treatment not working
- Seeing other people pregnant
- Google searches
- Something else?

Make a note of any that resonate with you. You will need them for the mindset tools in part two.

MY BIGGEST TRIGGERS

CHAPTER 3

A GROWING OBSESSION WITH GETTING PREGNANT

Everyone will experience different emotions on their journey. For me, the big ones were the total obsession about becoming pregnant, a crazy level of anxiety, endless worry about the future and, in general, a very negative mindset that got worse over time and became deep-rooted. Gone was my previous positive and sunny outlook, and in crept a very cynical and negative view on life, which seemed to consume me day in and day out.

Trying to get pregnant definitely brings out obsessive behaviour and it doesn't take long to become that way. I've known women trying to conceive for only a few months who say it's all they can think about and how frustrated they are. Fast-forward a few long months – and, very often, years – of trying, and these feelings only escalate.

When I think about someone who is obsessed, characters like Glenn Close in the movie *Fatal Attraction* spring to mind – a slightly bonkers seductress who on the surface seemed charming, but on the inside was consumed with a growing obsession that led to her behaviour spiralling out of control, with devastating consequences. Okay, that might be an extreme comparison, but when I was trying to fall pregnant I could certainly relate to those obsessional tendencies, all simmering beneath the surface, coupled with an angry mindset I felt I couldn't control. I walked around with the mask on, pretending I was happy and enjoying life, and the next minute I was in the toilet checking my knickers for signs of blood and analysing every twinge in my tummy.

The signs I was obsessed – my list!

As my quest to get pregnant dominated my life and my thoughts more and more, I developed several secret daily rituals. I can only explain them as obsessive habits that I did on a very regular basis. And, of course, I didn't tell anyone about them – that was far too embarrassing! They were things I did on my own. I was too ashamed to admit them to anyone, not even my husband, and I couldn't believe that anyone else would be crazy enough to do them too!

As promised, here is my list. I'm going public with it now! Thankfully, I've since realized that I'm not the only one who has confessed to doing such things, so it's not quite as embarrassing or shameful as I originally thought!

Read the list below and consider your own behaviour. How many of these rituals have you caught yourself doing since you've been trying to get pregnant? And how often... monthly, weekly or even daily?

- Googling "early pregnancy symptoms" repeatedly until I found the same symptom I had
- Doing pregnancy tests every month, far too early
- Prodding my boobs constantly whenever I was on my own, to see if they were swollen or sore
- Cancelling social functions in case I was pregnant
- Avoiding booking holidays in case I was pregnant
- Smiling and saying congratulations when people told me they were pregnant, but then going home and crying
- Avoiding friends who were pregnant
- Avoiding social events with families

- Googling "unexplained infertility success stories" and looking for a tenuous link to my situation
- Going to see mediums or Tarot readers to cling to some hope that I might get pregnant
- Spending loads of money on endless alternative therapies including reflexology, acupuncture and Chinese herbs
- Buying every book going about fertility
- Buying every multivitamin going for fertility
- Cutting out caffeine and alcohol because it affected fertility (I even cut out chocolate for a year because it contained caffeine, totally crazy!)
- Beating myself up with negative self-talk because I wasn't pregnant and might never be

It's exhausting reading that list, almost as much as it was hiding all those behaviours. I felt like two different people – the calm, together person on the outside and the obsessive, crazy one on the inside. I've since learnt that lots of people obsess about pregnancy in exactly the same way, and I'm sure you can identify with a few of those behaviours yourself.

CHAPTER 4

DOUBLE HELPINGS OF ANXIETY

While I was on my fertility journey, I was in a constant state of anxiety. My life was on hold until I got pregnant, and my happiness depended on it.

When you are feeling anxious, your mind is in the future, not the present. You are consumed with worry about a future event, in this case not getting pregnant. People get anxious about all sorts of things. It might be a fear of heights or a fear of flying. It could be a significant event, like a big presentation or a job interview or perhaps an upcoming sporting challenge. This kind of anxiety is event-specific, so it comes and goes. However, people still get physical symptoms when they are anxious, even for a short time, whether that be a churning stomach, shaking hands, a headache or even a full-blown panic attack.

My anxiety was constant, and my worries were overwhelming. The pattern of daily thoughts that would run through my mind would go something like this…

Am I pregnant? Is that an early pregnancy sign? Can I still book my holiday next year? Why aren't I getting pregnant? Why is this happening to me? Why does everyone else get pregnant so easily? What's wrong with me? What will life be like if I don't get pregnant? How will I juggle fertility treatments with work? What if it never happens to me? And what will I do when the money runs out?!

It makes me anxious just reading that!

With this level of constant anxiety, it's not difficult to imagine how much it must have affected my body without me even realizing it. When you're anxious, your mind is running at 100 miles per hour with negative chatter, rather than being calm and still. My stress levels must have been elevated on a pretty regular basis, and it's been medically proven that stress can affect the delicate balance of hormones – not at all helpful when you are trying to create the perfect monthly cycle!

Thoughts become things... the wrong things!

The other problem with my anxiety was that all the thoughts that consumed me were about things I didn't want to happen, rather than what I was really hoping for! People have a natural tendency to think about what might go wrong in life, instead of what might go right – crazy, eh? If we've got a job interview, we tend to immediately think, "What if I mess it up?" If we try out a new hobby, we might think we won't be any good at it. If we want to ask the boss for a pay rise, we automatically think they will never go for it. For some reason, it's easier to envision a negative outcome than it is to think about a more positive one. Think, "What if the boss says yes to that pay rise? What if I love that new hobby? And what if I breeze through the interview and get the job of my dreams?!"

This pattern of negative thinking was a huge problem I discovered in my quest to become pregnant. I spent 80% of my day thinking about all the things that I didn't want to happen – not getting pregnant, not being a mother, a life without children, feeling so alone. Many people have written about the Law of Attraction and the belief that what we think about is what we attract in our life, and I could see this unfolding in my own life quite clearly. If you're going about your day visualizing what you don't want, it's no surprise that nothing changes and you end up creating more of the same.

Think about it. Are you a glass-half-full or glass-half-empty kind of person? Do you go for that interview thinking that you won't get the job? Do you make excuses not to do something new for fear of failure? Do you tend to expect the worst in life and find you're usually proven right? If that's you, don't panic just yet. You might have fallen into this pattern of thinking when you weren't getting pregnant, but rest assured, even the most positive people have negative thoughts at times, and that's okay. The problem arises when your negative thoughts become your dominant way of thinking for most of the time.

CHAPTER 5

OVERTHINKING EVERYTHING

The other problem with anxiety is that it starts to consume your thoughts. When your mind is running wild all day with anxious thoughts about when and how you are going to get pregnant, it's hard to separate these thoughts from who we really are underneath all that. Over time, these thoughts can become so automatic and so intense, they become our reality – we become what we think about, and we believe what we think, even if it isn't true! This is often when depression can set in. Have you ever woken up in the morning feeling happy and rested, and then almost immediately, *wham*... the enormity of your fertility struggle hits you while you're lying in bed? Those thoughts escalate, and a cloud of depression appears that can stay with you for the rest of the day.

Having these thoughts first thing in the morning creates negative feelings and behaviours that end up dominating the day. When I was living my life constantly worrying about the future without a baby, I felt as though I was permanently walking around under a cloud. I found it so hard to appreciate everything else in my life, or see any good in it, because this one goal of trying to get pregnant dominated everything.

In this situation, it's good to remind yourself that any thoughts you have are only in your head. They're not real and they're not who you are. You choose how you think about any situation in your life – in this case, whether you get pregnant or not. You have the power to choose whether or not you look at what's happening to you with a positive, open mind, or if you choose to take a more cynical and negative view.

A classic example would be the two-week wait. You might hear the little voice inside your head saying, "Well, of course you're not going to be pregnant this month," or, "It will never work for you." Yet again, you are focusing on what could go wrong, rather than what could go *right*. Remind yourself that any anxious thoughts you may have are not real. You cannot predict what will happen to you, you are just envisaging one possible outcome, and sadly, it is quite often the worst one!

Once you really get this, it can be quite a light-bulb moment, the realization that you create your own thoughts and that they are not real. In more basic terms, you're making these thoughts up all day long, every day. You choose what type of thoughts you apply to any situation in your life, so you may as well construct some more positive, beneficial thoughts that will help you on this journey, instead of hindering you.

Distracted with mental chatter

When I was anxious all the time, it prevented me from living my life in the present moment. I lived my life worrying about a future without children, or a fear of not being able to get pregnant, and an overwhelming anxiety about what on earth was wrong with me. The mental chatter was so constant that I was nowhere near being present, or "mindful", as people refer to it these days. There is a huge amount written about the benefits of mindfulness and the ability to keep our minds in the present moment. If you think about it, there are no problems in the present moment – it's just what is happening around us right now. According to many self-help gurus, practising being in the present moment and focusing on what is going on right now is the key to happiness. Many people say that problems are created by how we think about an experience in our lives, rather than the experience itself – an interesting perspective.

Therefore, if we can avoid dwelling on things that have already happened, or worrying about things that have yet to happen, we can focus our attention on the present moment as much as possible. Looking back now I can clearly see that my mind was all over the place while I was trying to conceive. I was in a constant state of anxiety, and I was as far away from mindful as I could get!

Think about a time when you felt really happy, or you were really enjoying yourself. It could be something big, like a holiday or a special event you went to. Or perhaps it was something more routine, like spending time with good friends, doing a hobby that you love or simply enjoying a hot bath. Whatever it was, try to recall where your mind was at that time. When you are really happy, time tends to stand still. Chances are that when you were enjoying yourself, you weren't thinking about the past, or worrying about the future or any problems you might have. You were simply enjoying the present moment and what was going on right then, and it felt good… really good.

Anxiety tends to be focused on worries about future events, whereas depression often relates to past events from which we can't move on. Neither of these mindsets allows us to be in the present moment, and on a fertility journey it's so common to feel distracted like this. If we can learn how to reduce these anxious thoughts and train our minds to focus on the present moment, even if just for short periods of time, this is where we can begin to find happiness again and start to regain control.

CHAPTER 6

STRUGGLING TO SEE YOURSELF PREGNANT

One question I always ask my clients is whether they can see themselves pregnant. The ability to visualize what you want in life is a powerful, science-based tool that can be used in all areas of life with huge benefits. There are many success stories out there from big names in sport and business, such as Richard Branson, Conor McGregor and the Williams sisters, to name but a few. The basic idea is that if you can visualize something you want in your life, you can undoubtedly achieve it. By focusing on what you want and creating a clear vision of success in your mind, you then start to believe you can achieve it, and you direct your behaviour and energy toward this goal. As a result, you will manifest this vision in your life.

It's easier to visualize something you believe in. For example, if you're buying a new house and the sale of your old house has given you the funds to buy the house of your dreams, then it's quite easy to get yourself focused on a positive end result. You're excited, you know it's going to happen, and it probably will. But throw in a few problems – maybe one house fell through, maybe you haven't got enough money to buy the type of house you want, or maybe you have a strict deadline to meet… It's a bit harder to visualize success, isn't it? Your mind very quickly pushes the problems to the forefront. Successful visualization means focusing on the end result instead of all the problems along the way, and it's the same with your baby goal.

In my case, I realized that I was walking around with a vision that was so far away from what I actually wanted. The images in my head were all linked to my worries about not getting pregnant. I was seeing myself disappointed about not getting pregnant, living my life without being a mum, being the only one who wasn't pregnant. This thinking was so automatic I didn't think I could control it. It was certainly dominating a lot of my day. As a result, these thoughts were what I manifested in my life and nothing was changing.

I have often found that clients find it difficult to visualize themselves pregnant, particularly if they have been on this journey for a while. Somehow, it's scary to open themselves up to this image, particularly after many disappointments. Often, they are protecting themselves in case of failure. This is totally understandable, but it is not helpful to their success. So, unlocking a clear image of you being successful with pregnancy is a critical first step to creating a more positive mindset, whether that's seeing yourself pregnant or seeing yourself as a mother.

Imagining a future you don't want

When you are feeling anxious about not getting pregnant, your thoughts will be creating a vision for an outcome you don't really want. For example, thoughts of "I can't get pregnant" will lead to a vision of you without a baby. The problem here is that the brain can't tell the difference between what's real and what isn't. It will simply respond to what you're thinking about. And that's not good if most of your thoughts are about not getting pregnant. If we have faith that we will get pregnant when the time is right, this creates more positive images, and therefore positive feelings and behaviours. If we constantly worry that we won't get pregnant, we get a very different set of feelings and behaviours. It's not easy to focus on the good stuff though, especially after months or years of disappointment.

To test out how powerful your imagination is, try this simple visualization exercise:

Close your eyes and hold your hands out in front of you. Imagine someone has placed a freshly cut lemon in your hands. Picture the lemon right in front of you and start to smell it. Then, imagine yourself picking up that lemon and taking a huge bite out of the flesh. Imagine the bitter taste of the lemon and feel the juice bursting into your mouth. Is your mouth starting to water yet? Are you swallowing more than normal?

It's a simple exercise but it shows you how easily the brain and body respond to your vivid imagination. There is no lemon, of course, but the brain still responds as if there is!

As I said, when you are worrying all the time about not getting pregnant and what life will be like without a baby, your brain and body will start responding to these images. You might see this in how you're feeling. I regularly felt depressed, stressed and just generally sad. Physically, my body often felt tired. I found my energy levels were a lot lower than normal and I sometimes noticed subtle changes in my cycle.

The other problem is that feelings dictate your behaviour. When you are feeling good, you tend to behave more positively. You take more action and get things done. You can push or challenge yourself, and you are much more relaxed and open minded to new ideas.

Similarly, when you are feeling down, this also affects your behaviour. As such, if you're feeling depressed, sad or tired, it's going to be a bit of an effort to keep yourself fit and healthy, or take the practical steps you need to get pregnant. You might miss new opportunities around you that could take you closer to your goal of getting pregnant. You might be generally more negative or defensive, and you might hear yourself making excuses not to do things, especially if they're out of your comfort zone – and all this from some anxious thoughts YOU created in your imagination.

Good day or bad day?

Have you ever had a day when you wake up on top form? You spring out of bed and right away you're on fire, getting things done and achieving LOADS very easily. You're happier, calmer, less likely to react negatively and more likely to overcome any obstacles. Alternatively, when you have a bad day, you take ages to get going, you procrastinate, you avoid anything difficult, you drift through the day with low energy, and problems seem overwhelming.

How you wake up and what you do first thing in the morning sets your tone for the entire day. It's so important to give yourself a moment to create the mindset you want to keep for the rest of the day. You might wake up in a cloud of depression when you realize you've been trying for a baby for over a year, but there are things you can do to shift that mindset – simple, easy steps that work. But more about that later.

CHAPTER 7

AVOIDING TAKING ACTION

One of the biggest side effects of having a Fertility Mindset Meltdown is that it will stop you from taking action toward your goal of getting pregnant, without you even realizing it.

There is a great saying that sums this up perfectly, "If you always do what you've always done, you'll always get what you've always got". Or another way of putting it – nothing changes if nothing changes.

To create change in any area of your life, you first have to take action. You must do something different to change the situation, however small that first step may be. But whether or not you take action is often linked to how you feel on a particular day. How many of us join a gym with great intentions, but then find after a month we don't feel like going anymore? Reality check here – you may never feel like going to the gym! But people who are successful take action anyway and will go to the gym even when they don't feel like it because they know that it benefits them!

It's the same with your fertility journey. When you're feeling depressed, negative, sad or anxious, it's hard to find the energy to get out there and take action with your fertility plan. You might not have the energy to take the steps you need to – it may seem too overwhelming. When you come across obstacles, or have a medical setback, it's all too easy to give up. Perhaps you hear yourself making excuses. I used to do that a lot. I'd hear myself saying things like, "That treatment will never work for me," or, "My situation is different so I'm not trying that," or, "That's too expensive, I can't do that." My mindset became very fixed and as a result I missed opportunities around me – big things, like new treatment options, and small ones, like friends' suggestions or new ideas I would read about but not pay much attention to.

When you feel overwhelmed, helpless and out of control, often that can stop you from acting. But taking regular action is one of the most important steps to getting pregnant. So many of my clients came to me at the point when they were drifting through their fertility journey. They were simply waiting for something different to happen or hoping for a different result each month, rather than taking control, going out there and making it happen. As a result, the weeks, months and often years were drifting by and still they weren't pregnant.

I cannot stress enough how important action is on this journey. Taking small, practical steps forward will take you closer toward your goal of getting pregnant. It will mean you are exploring all opportunities, leaving no stone unturned and stopping at nothing to achieve your goal! Being motivated to take action requires a shift in your mindset. You have to want to do it. And that comes back to what's going on in your head and how your thoughts make you feel.

CHAPTER 8

FEELING LIKE TIME IS RUNNING OUT

When I was 15 years old, one of my oldest friends and I hatched a plan for the future. We decided that we would meet up in our home town when we were 25, with all our kids in tow, and reminisce about being young! Well, 25 came and went, and I didn't even have a husband, let alone children. And I was still living in my home town – disaster!

Tick-tock, the biological clock

Isn't it funny how we create a certain order of how we think things should happen in our lives, and by when? You might have wanted to move out of your parents' home by the time you were 22, get married and buy a house by 25 and, of course, have kids by the time you were 30! I'm not quite sure who decides on the timeline, and it will vary for different people, but let's admit it, we all had one.

It could be our parents' influence, or society's view on the order and timing of how people should do things, but one thing's for sure – it certainly adds an element of pressure. My mum finally had me when she was 28, after trying for 5 years to get there. Back in the 70s, being a first-time mum at the age of 28 was positively ancient. But now, 50 years later, times have changed, and 28 seems quite young – too young almost! These days many women get pregnant a bit later, wanting to enjoy their lives and careers first before settling down. When I was working with clients who were on a fertility journey, they all had one thing in common – they wanted to be pregnant before they hit 40. I was exactly the same. What is it about 40 that is such a big milestone? As you go through your 30s it looms over you like a big black cloud. Perhaps it's because, from a medical perspective, being 40 is associated with a fertility drop. There are so many statistics out there to say that after 40 your egg supply depletes, the quality of your eggs lowers, and therefore it gets much harder to become pregnant. When you're trying to get pregnant and reading this everywhere, it is inevitable that it will affect your mindset and create a subconscious "deadline" in your head.

When I was at the fertility clinic and discussing my chances of IVF success, I was always quoted all the average statistics, which meant that as I was approaching 40, my age was working against me. I was told many times that at my age, statistically, my chances of IVF success were very low. But when I sat in the waiting room chatting to the other women going through the same process, it was far from an average story. The room was full of women of all ages with a vast array of stories to tell. I remember one woman in her late 20s, supposedly a highly fertile age, who had been stimulated with fertility drugs and was struggling to produce any eggs at all. And there were other women approaching 40 going into the egg removal with swollen tummies because they had overstimulated and were producing too many eggs. I can remember one woman who was a similar age to me being told she was responding to the drugs like a 20-year-old, and then another younger girl being desperately upset as she had lots of eggs, but none were of good enough quality to be removed. The fact was, everyone had a different experience and not many were in line with the average. There are so many individual reasons behind people's infertility, and yet when you go into an IVF clinic, your chances of success are still compared to the "average" statistics for your age.

The truth is that lots of women get pregnant in their 40s very easily – in fact, a close friend of mine's sister got pregnant by accident at 49 when she thought she was going through the menopause! When you're on a fertility journey and you have your 40th birthday looming in front of you, it's so important to find a way to remove this invisible barrier from your head. It can also be harder if you are a control freak planner like me and want everything to be perfect. Instead, you need to practise being open to things happening slightly differently to the way you had first imagined. You might get pregnant at a different age, possibly later than you had planned, but that's okay. See what you can do to remove this self-imposed deadline and avoid putting unnecessary pressure on your already tough journey.

Everything happens at the right time... in the end

Hindsight is a wonderful thing. When I look back now at my fertility journey, getting pregnant at 40 with triplets was so far from my original plan. If someone had told me at 30 that it would take me 10 years to have a baby, I would have been on the floor with desperation. But looking back now, although it was an extremely upsetting journey, in the end it has all worked out perfectly. If I had got pregnant when I started trying at 30, I have no doubt my first marriage would still have crumbled, and that would have impacted my children. If we had divorced, I would have had to share the kids with my ex-husband, and he would have been a regular part of my life. I may not have ever met Rob if I'd had kids and he didn't. My career wouldn't have reached the heights it did before I finally had a family, meaning I had much more experience to fall back on when I started working again. And we may not have found our dream house if we'd had kids earlier. The year before I finally got pregnant, we embarked on a huge renovation project that would never been a priority with young kids in tow!

I had always wanted more than one child so, in fact, having triplets meant that I caught up with everyone in one go. My ready-made family arrived in one perfect bundle, and I only had to go through one pregnancy. We were also more financially stable at 40 than we were in our 30s, and we'd had years to get the free time and partying out of our systems.

Looking back at all of that now, even though it didn't feel like it at the time, in the end the timing was just right.

My fertility journey has definitely taught me the power of patience and to be open to the fact that things may happen in a slightly different way to how you first plan them. But in the end, you can still get there. Being a new mum in my early 40s seemed old to me at first, but there are a lot of benefits. I'm definitely older and wiser! They say your worst nightmare can become your biggest opportunity, and it's the tough times in life that give you the chance to grow and learn. I believe that I'm a better person for everything I went through on my ten-year fertility journey, and I can only hope that some of my resilience and positivity will rub off on our children.

Exercise: Your timeline of events

Have a think about your own timeline of events, using these questions:

- What timeline of events are you holding on to?

- What's driving that timeline?

- What's important to you about things happening that way?

- How can you let go of that timeline and be open to something new?

- How could a different timeline look?

- What would happen if getting pregnant takes a few years longer than you thought it would?

- What benefits are there for things happening later?

Look objectively at your timelines and try and be open to things happening in different ways. Question and challenge yourself about why your original timeline is so important to you and what is really driving it. Try and reframe the situation and consider how things could happen in a different way. Think back to other areas of your life where events happened at a different time to how you had originally planned – did it all work out in the end?

Use this exercise to try and reframe your own timeline for getting pregnant so that you are not putting extra pressure on yourself. Create a new timeline that feels okay and is realistic for you to work toward from where you are right now. Record your thoughts in the box on the next page.

MY IDEAL TIMELINE OF EVENTS	HOW THINGS COULD HAPPEN DIFFERENTLY – A NEW TIMELINE
What is driving this timeline?	What are the benefits of this timeline?

PART THREE

MINDSET TOOLS –
TAKE BACK CONTROL

I don't have a magic wand to get you pregnant. It will happen when it's supposed to happen, but I completely understand that not knowing when that will be is hugely frustrating. What I can do is help you take back control of your journey and give you the tools to transform what is going on in your head. These tools will help you remove all the emotional pain and overwhelming negativity that is dragging you down, and replace it with a new energy and joy in your life that ultimately gets your fertility journey back on track and moving in the right direction again. And when you feel more positive, you will take more action, which takes you closer to your goal of getting pregnant. Plus, you should feel much happier along the way.

CHAPTER 9

BE HAPPY NOW

The quest to be happy is a bit of a holy grail in life. Browse the self-help section of any good bookstore and you will likely see numerous books advertising the latest theory on how to find happiness. As we grow up, we are often taught that being successful leads to happiness, meaning that we will be happy when we have achieved certain things in life, like good grades at school, a successful career or getting on the property ladder. And, of course, we will also be happy when we have that baby. In fact, we think that our happiness depends on it, and quite often we can't appreciate the rest of our life without it.

But these days there is more and more written about the fact that happiness is a choice and that, in order to be successful in life and achieve whatever we want, we need to be happy first. When you're happy, you are in a positive and more open state of mind. You have clear goals that you believe in, you are less likely to be affected by setbacks, criticism and obstacles, and, most importantly, you have the energy and motivation to take action toward your goals.

Being happy first is just as important when you're trying to get pregnant. Focusing on what's already good in your life and being grateful for what you have now will help bring more of it to you. Think about it: when you're happy, you feel good, and quite often more good things tend to happen. Once you appreciate that the thoughts you have in your head can be controlled, you begin to realize that happiness is very much a choice for you every day. You decide how you respond to the events that happen around you and how you think about them, which ultimately decides whether or not you are going to be happy that day. That doesn't mean you won't have setbacks and feel down when things go wrong. That's part of life, and just like the Yin needs the Yang, you can't experience joy in your life without some understanding of pain. But when you're happy, you bounce back quicker, you don't let things affect you long term, and you know what you need to do to pick yourself up after disappointments and get back on track.

This section contains some of the tools I used – and continue to use – to help me be happy in the present. Once I realized that my mindset was working against me on my pregnancy journey, I wanted to retrain my thoughts to calm my mental chatter, and keep me as present and positive as possible. There was a lot of trial and error, but here's what worked for me.

CHAPTER 10

COMMIT TO DAILY MINDSET TRAINING

Being happy every day might seem like a simple choice but, when you are stuck in negative patterns of thinking, it can be hard to break this cycle and start the day a different way. Making that change starts with a commitment to training your mind to think differently. Just like signing up for a gym programme to train your muscles, you can commit to some daily mindset training to tackle what's going on in your head.

The mindset tools in this chapter will provide a daily routine to help you train your mind to work with you on this journey and keep you focused on where you want to be (a mum with a family), and not where you don't want to be (living a life without children). Research shows that people tend to think more negative thoughts than positive thoughts about any situation in life, and when you've been on a fertility journey for a while, it may feel like you are automatically thinking more pessimistically about your outlook.

Remember that the mind is like a muscle, and with regular and consistent effort, it can be trained to think in a more positive way. Although these mindset tools are simple, as with any new routine, you need to put the effort in to keep them up, especially at the start. These negative patterns of thinking have built up over time, and breaking the cycle requires commitment and a consistent daily routine until they become a more automatic way of thinking.

To build a new routine into your life will likely require trial and error at first. I'm a big believer in making regular small changes rather than changing everything all at once, which can be impossible to stick to in the long term. It's like the classic January ritual of embarking on a new fitness regime. We announce to the world that we will be training five days a week, going on strict diets and not drinking any alcohol. What usually happens (to me anyway) is that I give it my all for a couple of weeks, but then it's just too hard to stick to, so I come rolling off the wagon and beat myself up for not having the discipline to go the distance.

Small steps lead to big changes

What's much more realistic and effective long term is committing to some small changes that you can make regularly and consistently. Think about the flight plan that an aircraft follows. If the plane is just one degree off course, its trajectory may not look very different at first, but it makes a huge difference to where the plane ends up landing. It's the same with the changes you make for yourself. If you make just one small degree of change today and stick to that change consistently, it will have a massive impact on your outcome in the long run.

Work out how you can build these tools into the pockets of your life. Find times in the day that work for you. Chances are, you will launch into your new routine enthusiastically for the first couple of weeks, and then you might relax a bit and start to miss days, especially if you aren't seeing results. Be patient and don't give up too soon. Doing this work is like planting a seed. If you plant a seed, it can take a bit of time for it to germinate and flower, and it needs feeding and nurturing along the way. In the same way, it will take time for you to get into a routine and see your results. Practising these tools daily is like feeding and nurturing your seed. You don't turn around after three days and say, "Well, that's not working," and give up. You commit to looking after your seed each day and before long you might see a bud pop through, giving you the motivation to continue. Look out for any signs that your new tools are working, however small. Be open and notice the positive changes or opportunities that start to present themselves.

Once you've got a routine that works for you, I would suggest starting with a consistent daily practice for a period of 21 days. This is the proven length of time to create a new habit, and in this case, a new pattern of thinking. Make a 21-day commitment to invest time in YOU and get your fertility journey back on track.

If you miss a day, don't beat yourself up, just get straight back into it the next day. Remind yourself how important this is, how things weren't working before and that change is needed. Before long, you will notice that your new routine comes much more easily to you, and that's how new habits are formed.

I would also recommend buying a journal or notebook where you can record your thoughts and the exercises. It's a good place to keep track of highlights as a reminder, and you can look back on your progress. Treat yourself and buy a really special notebook that is just for you.

CHAPTER 11

CREATE A POSITIVE MORNING ROUTINE

How you wake up and start your day is critical to how the rest of the day unfolds. Think about your morning routine. What happens from the second you wake up? When you are lying in bed and trying to drag yourself up, what are you thinking about? When you're going through your normal morning routine, whether that's in the bathroom, getting dressed or having breakfast, what kind of things affect your mood?

When you are facing problems in life, it's quite common to wake up feeling relaxed and calm in your bed, and then, moments later, all that changes when the enormity of your situation hits you. Once again you have woken up and you're still not pregnant. You have no idea whether or not it will happen. You start worrying about the future; the anxiety kicks in and immediately that sets a bad tone for the day.

Phones have also become a detriment to morning routines. Perhaps you wake up and immediately reach for the phone. Suddenly you are connected to the outside world straight away through emails, messages and, of course, social media. It's not even 7am, and you are already comparing yourself to the seemingly perfect families online! You also check emails and instantly start worrying about your to-do list. You have a constant ping of messages to reply to, and so your day begins in this slightly frantic way.

Quite often your morning routine is on autopilot. You probably get up the same way you have done for years: wake up, check your phone, start worrying about your to-do list, make coffee, get dressed. You might rush because you laid in bed too long, and that means you could start snapping at your partner because you're late. You're distracted with what you have to do that day, which means you are far from present. Finally, you get in the car, and how are you feeling then? Tired, grumpy, depressed and slightly stressed. It's not the best start to the day, but you just carry on and then repeat it all the next morning!

Win the first hour, win the day

It's a slightly cheesy expression, but I really like the meaning behind it. If you can create a more positive start to your day, first thing in the morning, you will start to see a positive impact on the rest of your day. I would like you to commit to starting your day differently, every day. It's not going to take you long, but a few small tweaks to your morning routine can make a big difference to your day. Creating a few minutes to follow a short mindset routine first thing in the morning can have a hugely positive impact, and it's something you can revisit at key points throughout the day, whenever you need a quick reset or a mental boost.

I created a morning routine that worked for me. It was short, simple and easy to build into my day. I practised it whenever I had moments to myself, and over time I noticed a huge shift in my mindset, including a difference in how I responded to challenges when they came along. I also noticed my mindset slipping again if I skipped the routine for a while. I realized that by doing the routine for just a few minutes each day, it had a hugely positive impact on how I felt that day, and therefore how I behaved. Read on to find out more…

CHAPTER 12

ADOPT AN ATTITUDE OF GRATITUDE

Are you grateful for what is in your life right now? Okay, you're not pregnant, and I know that is the most important thing to you, but do you appreciate everything you *do* have? I saw a fantastic quote online once that said, "You may not be living your dream yet, but you're living someone else's right now." It definitely makes you think. You might not have the baby you want but look at what you do have. Perhaps you're in a happy, loving relationship. You might have a house, a good job, regular income, or good friends and family around you. You might be blessed with good health and have the opportunity to go places and travel. And at a very basic level, you have a roof over your head, you have food, and you have your freedom. When you're on this very tough journey, it's easy to take for granted what you already have in your life, as wanting a baby is the only thing on your mind.

Research into gratitude shows that grateful people are happier and healthier. When you're not getting pregnant and having constant setbacks, even the most positive person can switch from a glass-half-full to a glass-half-empty outlook. Rather than focusing on all the good stuff you do have, you focus on the one thing you don't. When you're grateful every day, it creates a positive energy around you and helps you see life more optimistically. Being truly grateful makes you feel good too. It makes you feel happier and, according to the Law of Attraction, when you're grateful you will attract more things to be grateful for. That works the other way too: when you're anxious you will attract more things to be anxious about.

Think about it – when something goes wrong, do you fear the worst? And is your inner chatter during the day full of what's wrong with your world, rather than what's right with it?

The universe loves grateful people, and if you're grateful every day, you will start to see things more positively. You'll notice a shift in the way you respond to events around you, and as a result you may see more good things coming into your life. Gratitude is a multiplier, so be grateful for everything positive in your life, however small.

Once you commit to being grateful every day, it will become easier the more you do it. Quite soon, you will automatically start to have a more positive and grateful response to what's happening in your life. Try it and wait for the magic to start.

What are you grateful for right now?

In your journal, write a list of things to be grateful for about your fertility journey so far. Okay, so you're not pregnant yet, and that's what you ultimately want to happen, but what are the positive aspects of it all? If you've waited two years and still haven't had a baby, what have you been able to do in that time that you couldn't have done if you were pregnant? Move house? Travel abroad? Or if you've had a failed treatment, what were the positive things that happened along the way? Maybe you responded well to the drugs, perhaps you were able to freeze some eggs? It may not be easy to do this at first, but it really does help. It's all part of the process to retrain your mind to see the good stuff rather than blocking it out and focusing on what's going wrong.

Once you have your list, look back on it regularly, especially on the bad days. Remind yourself that everything happens at the right time in the end and be grateful for the positive aspects of your journey so far.

I'm not saying you need to be on a positive, grateful high 24/7. That would be rather annoying, I'm sure! Of course, bad days happen and, on this journey, you will face many setbacks and disappointments. But once you start to bounce back from a situation, try to make a conscious effort to be grateful for any positives that happened along the way. It will definitely help you recover more quickly and face the future more positively.

Daily gratitude

When you wake up first thing in the morning, focus on what's good in your life. Before you even get out of bed, give thanks for your cosy bed, a good night's sleep, your partner, your family, your health... whatever comes to mind. If it's helpful for you, write your gratitude down or use one of the many gratitude apps now available online. Identify a minimum of three things to be grateful for each day. I have a beautiful gratitude manual, and every day I write a list of what I'm thankful for; I've been doing it for about 15 years now. I'm a morning person, so I write it right when I get up, but if you're better in the evenings, you can do it before you go to bed. It's a lovely way to finish the day, and you can read it through again when you wake up to help reinforce the feeling of gratitude.

Being grateful is something you can do at any time in the day. You can practise gratitude lying in bed when you first wake up, while you're in the shower, while you're waiting for the kettle to boil, or even driving in your car – pretty much any time you have a moment to yourself. Try to do this fairly early on in your day if you can. It only takes a few minutes to think about what you're grateful for, and it's a much more positive way to start your day than stressing about what you have to do and whether or not you will be pregnant this month. You might think, "I haven't got time to do all that, I'm so busy!" but all I'm asking for is a few minutes every day as you go about your morning routine. It will help to reset your mindset each morning and replace the negative chatter you may not even realize is spinning round your head, which automatically sets a more negative tone for the day.

As the day goes on, look out for more things to be grateful for. If something positive happens, say "thank you"! It could be something major that happens in your life, like a new job or a promotion, or it could be a very small thing. If you get green lights all the way to work, be grateful for that just as much as you would be if you got a pay rise.

Say "thank you" to people as you go through the day, and don't forget to say it to your partner too. Watch how infectious it is. With my husband, I find that the more I thank him for doing things for me, the more he will do for me, which can be very handy (and that's why I'm always thanking him for putting the bins out!). People like to be appreciated in life, so it makes them feel good if you thank them for doing something. And if you're genuinely grateful for the people in your life, you will receive that gratitude back in bucketloads.

So often we have bad days and go to bed miserable about what happened, beating ourselves up about the latest events that didn't go our way – not a great way to fall asleep. Be thankful for something every day, especially on the bad days, last thing at night. Lie in bed and think of one good thing that happened in your day before you go to sleep – it will end things on a more positive note. Even now I do this with my kids. Every day before they go to sleep, I ask them what the best bit was about their day. We have a little chat, and it's a nice, positive way for them to fall asleep. It's become such a ritual that if I forget, they shout out as I'm walking out of the bedroom, "Mummy, you didn't do the best bit of the day!"

Feel grateful too

Some people have said to me, "Oh, but I've started the day with my three things to be grateful for, but nothing has changed in my life!" There are two things to say about this. Firstly, when you are writing your list, do you FEEL grateful for what you're writing about? It's the feeling of gratitude that creates the shift in your energy, so it's important that you really hook into that. Think about why you're grateful and that will help you appreciate the situation even more. Try this with just one thing you're truly grateful for. Why are you grateful for having this particular thing in your life? How does it make you feel? Focus on this feeling and make it is as powerful as it can be – feel it flowing round your body and tap into that energy for at least 15 seconds or more.

Secondly, are you grateful as you go through the rest of your day? It's no good doing five minutes of gratitude first thing in the morning and then spending the rest of the day taking everything for granted, complaining about life or feeling anxious about what's not going right. Commit to a regular practice of gratitude. Think of it as part of your daily mindset routine, and over time it will become a more automatic way or responding to your life. If you miss a day, don't beat yourself up at all, just get back on track the next day. Even if you don't have time to write it down, make a conscious effort to find things to be grateful for as you go through your day. My friend and I went through a stage of texting each other our three reasons for gratitude every morning. By doing this, we held each other more accountable and were much more likely to do it daily. It was also a really positive start to the day, and we both felt that it was a great way of keeping in touch with what was going on in one another's lives – and with all the positive stuff too, not just the moans and groans you might normally offload to your friends!

You can practise gratitude in the shower, or in the car, or wherever you have time to yourself. And don't forget to FEEL that you are grateful – that is so important. It might be difficult at first but after a while, if you are spending more time being grateful than not, you will start to respond this way more automatically and notice a positive shift in your life.

CHAPTER 13

REPLACE NEGATIVE BELIEFS WITH POSITIVE AFFIRMATIONS

When people think of affirmations, they quite often picture someone sitting cross-legged, meditating and repeating a mantra. "Total mumbo jumbo," you might say, or it may seem a bit far out and definitely not something that can easily be incorporated into a daily routine.

But if you think about it, your mind is full of affirmations all day long. Your internal chatter is going non-stop from the moment you get up to the time you go to bed, and quite often that includes statements (or affirmations) concerning your beliefs about yourself. These affirmations can be positive but quite often they can work against you. You might say in the mornings, "I'm stressed," "I'm going to be late," or, "I'm rubbish at my job." Or if you suffer a disappointment one day, you might say, "Well, that was always going to happen to me," or, "Things always go wrong for me." And if you have something important to do one day, you might tell yourself, "This isn't going to go well, I'm going to fail at this." These statements are all affirmations – just negative, unhelpful ones. Instead of helping you, they are cementing the negative beliefs you have about yourself.

When you are on a fertility journey, you may not even realize that all day long, you are giving yourself a hard time, saying things like, "Getting pregnant will never happen to me," "I don't deserve a baby," "Everyone else gets pregnant except me," "I am always the unlucky one," and more! Your day is full of triggers that switch on this thinking, whether that's seeing someone else pregnant, getting your period (again) or having a failed treatment.

If these statements fill your head every day, they will start to influence how you feel and behave, and therefore what happens to you on your fertility journey. As you will already have read in Chapter 3, what you focus on grows over time, and when you continue to think these negative affirmations each day, they will become a self-fulfilling prophecy in your life. You won't have the energy to take the action you need to, you may stop believing that this can happen for you, and you will start to miss opportunities around you. Before you know it, you are drifting through your fertility journey with nothing changing and the weeks and months flying by.

Become an observer

The first step to changing this chatter is to start observing your thoughts and noticing what you are saying to yourself each day. Try looking for some patterns. What statements are you telling yourself that are limiting your potential? Listen hard – the voice inside you can be small but have a lot of power. What are the daily triggers for all your negative chatter? You can refer to your notes on this from Chapter 2. Are there any specific events or experiences that set off a particular pattern of thinking for you? Write down what you notice, when you notice it. Make a note on your phone if you are out and about as, believe me, you will forget it later. Becoming more self-aware and observing what's going on in your head is the first step to start changing things.

When you notice the negative chatter that goes on in your head and the limiting beliefs you are forcing on yourself, it can be quite shocking. I started to write down some of my daily thoughts and I was horrified. How could I be so critical of myself? How did this happen so automatically and seem so out of my control?

I also noticed how many thoughts my brain made up that really weren't true! How did I know I would never be pregnant? Was there really no one else out there who couldn't get pregnant except me? And who said I didn't deserve a baby? This was a bit of a light-bulb moment for me. Once I started to challenge the thoughts that I was having, I realized that a lot of the chatter and affirmations were completely unwarranted. They weren't factual in any way. They were just thoughts and statements that my brain had created, and I realized I could train my brain to create thoughts that were more positive.

Creating affirmations

Getting control of this negative chatter isn't easy at first. Goodness knows we all have it, in all areas of our life, and for some of us it may be the habit of a lifetime. Over time, these self-imposed beliefs can lead to all sorts of anxiety and depression. People may turn to counselling and start to dig deeply into why they are thinking in this way. This can be helpful in starting to challenge the thoughts you have, but it doesn't always work. My personal experience of counselling is that it is invaluable in some situations, particularly where there are deep-rooted issues that you need to work through. However, you need to find the right type of counselling that works for you – and the right counsellor. I have had some fantastic ones in the past, but I have also had some experiences that didn't feel helpful at all. In fact, some caused even more overthinking about my fertility issue, and therefore even more anxiety!

I discovered a really simple way to change your self-talk and feel more positive about your fertility through using positive affirmations. We know that our current patterns of thinking are based on our life experiences, from how we were brought up through to our adult experiences today. They can be deep-rooted and might seem so automatic that we think they can't possibly be changed. But they can. Any negative patterns of thinking have been created by us thinking in the same way repeatedly, over a long period of time. This becomes our default automatic response. Thankfully, we can create exactly the same process but with a more positive thought pattern instead.

We already know that the mind is like a muscle that can be trained to operate in a certain way. This means it is totally possible to retrain the chatter in your head in order to make it work *for* you, not against you. Some people choose to do this through counselling, and a deep analysis and challenge of each negative thought. This allows them to reframe the situation and think differently, which can definitely be helpful for a lot of people. For me personally, I found that working on my affirmations was a lot simpler and didn't require any more self-analysis – let's face it, on this journey, there's already enough of that!

Daily positive affirmations

When you identify the negative beliefs you are imposing on yourself each day, you can flip them into positive affirmations to replace them. These new positive affirmations will become your daily mantras, and you will repeat them regularly throughout the day, the idea being that you can retrain your mind to accept these new statements.

For example, if you subconsciously tell yourself daily, "I will never get pregnant," you could replace that with, "I am ready to be pregnant." Or if you often think "There's something wrong with me because I can't get pregnant," you could change that to, "I am perfectly healthy and ready to conceive."

The list below shows some typical negative statements that you may be thinking to yourself while trying to conceive. I have listed some suggested affirmations that you could flip them to, but please don't be restricted to my list – it's just a suggestion to get you going. It's really important that you identify your own self-limiting beliefs and flip them into positive affirmations that work for you. You might find that your affirmations apply to your life generally, not just to trying to conceive, but they are still impacting your fertility journey.

Common negative beliefs with suggested affirmations

NEGATIVE BELIEFS	SUGGESTED AFFIRMATIONS
I will never get pregnant.	My baby is on the way.
I have lost faith that this will happen to me.	I am happy now and ready to conceive.
There's something wrong with me.	I am perfectly healthy and ready to conceive.
Everyone else gets pregnant except me.	I deserve to be pregnant; I am ready to conceive.
I don't want a life without a baby.	I have a happy and fulfilling life; I love my life.
I don't deserve to be pregnant.	I deserve my baby and I'm ready to conceive.
I want to be pregnant before I'm 40.	I am pregnant at the right time for me.
I feel depressed about not being pregnant.	I feel excited and happy to be pregnant.
I feel anxious about the future.	I feel happy and excited about being a mum.
I worry too much.	I am relaxed and happy in the present moment.

(Continued)

NEGATIVE BELIEFS	SUGGESTED AFFIRMATIONS
I worry about the future.	I feel relaxed and excited about the future.
I am not good enough for this.	I am good enough just as I am.
Bad stuff always happens to me.	I deserve the very best in life and I accept it now.
I have always failed at this.	I am perfectly healthy and I can do this.
I am different, or not as good as everyone else.	I am good enough to achieve anything I want to.

Exercise: Your beliefs and affirmations

Now consider your own negative beliefs. What are the negative statements you find yourself thinking? How are you critical about yourself? How do you see yourself compared to others? Look back at your journal for any clues or notes you have observed.

Write a list of the negative beliefs or internal chatter that you have observed in yourself. Then, consider how you can flip these beliefs into a new, more positive affirmation.

It's important that your affirmation is written positively and in the present tense. This helps you feel like it's happening now. If it's in the future tense, you are affirming it's in the future – in other words, just out of reach – which is not where we want to put it. It also needs to be full of positive language. For example, "I don't want to feel anxious" would not be a good affirmation. The brain only hears the "anxious" part and as a result you are reinforcing what you don't want to happen. It would be much better to say something like, "I feel happy and excited about being a mum." Focus on the outcome you want, not what you don't want.

Record your thoughts in the table below.

MY NEGATIVE BELIEFS	NEW POSITIVE AFFIRMATIONS

Repeat, repeat, repeat!

Pick one or two affirmations that really work for you to help you transform your negative beliefs. The aim is to retrain your brain and replace the old negative statements with these new powerful affirmations.

When you first wake up and you're lying in bed, you can silently repeat your affirmation a few times. Feel, as deeply as you can, what it is like to believe that statement. It is hugely important to hook into the feeling that accompanies the affirmation. When you go to the bathroom and look at yourself in the mirror, you can repeat the affirmation again. It might even help to say it out loud when you look in the mirror. This might feel silly at first or make you feel self-conscious, but it is really powerful. Your physical response when you say your affirmation while looking at yourself might hint to whether you believe it or not. If you keep doing this daily, it will get easier to believe the new statement, and you will start to see this in your reaction.

Keep your affirmations going throughout the day, whenever you have time to yourself – in the shower, on the loo, waiting in a queue, walking, running, doing any kind of exercise. This might seem a bit out there, but remember that you are trying to replace the negative affirmations that already run through your head hundreds of times a day! Remind yourself that you are already thinking these affirmations all day long, but now you are replacing them with much more positive statements that will help you on this journey.

Visual cues

Set up visual cues to remind you to think about your affirmations. Write them in the front of your journal. Stick them on a Post-it note on the fridge, or on the bathroom mirror. Create a screensaver with them on it. Use a word from one as a password. One of my best friends changed their password to "Pregnant42" to reinforce her desired pregnancy and the age at which she wanted it to happen. Anything you can do to cement this affirmation during your day will really help you to start to believe it, and visual props are very powerful. Be creative and have some fun with it. Don't worry about what other people think, and remember that everyone has their own affirmations in their heads – you are just taking positive and more visual steps to create the change you need.

When you say your affirmation, start to think about how it would feel if the statement was true. This might be hard at first, and you might notice your internal chatter come flying back in with the perfect argument against it! Something like: "That's nonsense, this will never happen to you!" But keep doing it, keep saying your affirmation regularly each day – over time, that negative chatter will fade, and you will start to feel differently.

Try out your new affirmations for 21 days and see what happens. This approach might seem a bit simplistic, but there is so much evidence to say that it works and, combined with gratitude and visualization, it worked for me. Over time, I felt more positive and got my hope back. I noticed that my default response to situations was becoming more positive and I just felt a little bit happier and more excited about the future. This meant I had a new energy and was more receptive to new ideas and opportunities around me. I had confidence again and I saw a shift in my thinking. Ultimately, that meant that I was taking more action toward my goal of getting pregnant.

CHAPTER 14

VISUALIZE YOURSELF PREGNANT

Our brains are creating images in our heads all the time. Think back to the child at school who was daydreaming out of the window in their own little world. Or when you drive home from work and can't remember the last ten minutes of your commute because you were lost in a world of thoughts. We are thinking all the time and creating images in our head as we go through our days.

As we learnt in Chapter 6, visualization is a tool used with great success in all areas of life, and there are many high-profile examples in the sporting and business worlds. An athlete will be at the top of their game when they have both the technical expertise and the strength of mindset to succeed. The boxer Mohammed Ali famously visualized himself standing in the ring as the champion, and he started out his career using positive affirmations, referring to himself as "the greatest" even before he became the champion. Footballer Wayne Rooney used to lie in bed the night before a match, visualizing himself scoring goals. Michael Phelps used mental rehearsal to reach his peak swimming performance, visualizing every intricate detail of him winning a race, from how the water felt to the sounds and sights around him, almost programming his brain to operate in the way that would win him the race.

It's easy to visualize success when you are feeling good but it's more difficult to do this when times are tough. The actor Jim Carrey has told the story about how, when he was a broke, struggling actor, he used to drive to look at the Hollywood sign every night and visualize directors liking his work, just to make himself feel better. He also wrote himself a cheque for $10 million for acting services rendered, dated December 1995, as a goal for his Hollywood success. Incredibly, just before Thanksgiving in 1995, he was offered the part in the movie *Dumb and Dumber*, for which he was paid $10 million.

When you are feeling unhappy with your current situation, it takes practice and effort to visualize the success you want. There is a natural tendency for the brain to immediately focus on what's going wrong and the barriers in front of you. The skill here is to be able to visualize the future you want and have faith that it's coming, even when things are tough. If you can imagine it, you can achieve it.

This is the same for your fertility journey. Can you visualize yourself pregnant? Can you see yourself as a mother with a family? If you've been trying to conceive for a while, it may be harder for you to see this image in your mind. When you have other goals in life, like trying to get a new job or finding a new house, it's a much less emotionally charged goal, and it's therefore easier for you to objectively see in your mind the outcome you want. For example, when you move house, you will start out with a vision of the type of house you want to live in. When you are moving jobs, you know the type of job you want to secure. Without these clear visions, it would be a very frustrating process – a bit like driving around in a car with no idea where your destination is. Having said that, trying to have a baby and wanting to be a mum holds much more emotion and is a critical life goal. The pain of not getting pregnant or having repeated disappointments can stop you from visualizing a successful outcome. It can become painful to think about something so important that is not happening, and you may feel you need to protect yourself by not imagining it at all.

Exercise: Your vision

Being able to visualize yourself pregnant and seeing yourself as a mum is a *critical* step in managing your mindset and getting your fertility plan back on track. What I'd like you to do is to spend some time creating a specific vision of the outcome you want. It's helpful to do this when you have some time to yourself, preferably somewhere you won't be disturbed and can sit for a few minutes with your eyes closed.

The first step is to allow yourself to think about the future you want as a mum. Think about what life might be like for you when you are pregnant, or when you are a mum. Identify a specific time in the future that excites you. This could be you being pregnant with a big bump, or it could be a specific moment, like seeing the growing baby on the ultrasound for the first time. It could be you at the point of giving birth, or a bit further on, pushing a buggy around the park. It might even be a specific event in the longer-term future, such as a specific family holiday, or a milestone birthday that you are celebrating with your children there too. It could also be something simple, like feeding your baby at your favourite coffee shop or watching your baby asleep in their cot. It doesn't matter what your image is, but it has to be something that is meaningful to you. Create an image in your head, built on a specific time in the future.

Make it a detailed image

Close your eyes and create an image in your head based on this specific future event. It's important to spend a few minutes getting this image really clear. The more detailed and specific the image is, the more real it will appear to be and the more you will connect to it emotionally. Spend some time creating all the detail in your vision by asking yourself the questions on the next page.

- Where are you in this image?
- Who is with you?
- What are you doing?
- What are you wearing?
- What are your surroundings?
- What is going on in the image around you?
- What can you hear? What can you see?
- How are you feeling in this image?
- What are you thinking?
- How is everyone else feeling? How can you tell?
- What are people saying?
- What is your body language? And everyone else's?

Having a clear, detailed vision is critical in making it real for you. It may not be easy at first – you might just feel blank, or you may struggle to build any detail with your image. This could be for a number of reasons. Perhaps you don't want to allow yourself to go there and think about this event when it's clearly not happening. Or perhaps it's too emotional and painful to think about the event because you haven't got it right now. The pain of not having your baby can be overwhelming, and imagining yourself as a mum can bring all these feelings of sadness to the surface. That is normal, and it is okay. In fact, it's good to get these feelings out and release them to make room for more positive ones. If you need a cry, have one. If you start feeling angry, sometimes having a good scream or beating a pillow can release that anger. You may want to talk to someone else afterwards to share your vision and how it made you feel. Doing any of these things will help you release that suppressed emotion which is good for your stress levels. Don't give up on your vision, keep working on it daily to create a clear image in your head. With practice, it will get easier.

If you get the images straight away – that's brilliant! Just like with any other project in your life, you are visualizing yourself being successful at it. This one is more emotional, but it works in exactly the same way. The next step is to tap into this vision on a daily basis so that your brain starts to see it as a reality for you. By doing this, your energy and behaviour will respond in the same way, taking you closer to that goal.

Daily work on your vision

A bit like with your affirmation, think about this vision whenever you have some quiet time to yourself. This can be first thing in the morning or last thing at night. You might want to envision it while you're still lying in bed, or while you're in the shower. I used to have a long journey to work, and instead of thinking about my huge to-do list, I would spend the first five or ten minutes of the journey tapping into my vision and repeating my affirmation. It helped to get me into a positive mindset where there was hope and possibility. The key is to imagine your vision like it's happening right now, rather than some point in the future. You need to feel how good it is to be pregnant and what it's like to be a mum, and to do that you have to allow yourself to get excited. If you can do this on a daily basis, those feelings of excitement and gratitude will grow, and your vision will become more of an achievable reality for you.

In the same way as with your affirmation, visual cues are hugely important. My vision was all about me being pregnant and having a big bump that everyone could see. You will laugh, but I printed out a picture of a pregnant lady in the kind of outfit I could see myself wearing, and I taped a happy, smiling photo of my face on the top of it. And then I put it on the fridge for all to see! This meant I was looking at it regularly throughout the day, and it would automatically make me smile and create a little bit of excitement inside me. It was also a source of conversation when people came round. We would have a joke about it, but it was reinforcing me seeing myself pregnant all the time. Even my sister, bless her, created a similar image of me in a photo frame by her bed so she was visualizing me pregnant too! And I did actually become pregnant just a few months later, just saying!

Find your own visual cue that works for you. You could manipulate your own photo like I did, or you could create a vision board with a selection of images that work for you – people, places or things that relate to your vision. Be as creative as you can to identify some visual prompts that work for you. Technology can help you massively here. There are some fantastic apps to create photos and images, so have some fun with it!

Meditate on your vision

Meditation can be very helpful in cementing your vision. You could spend as little as five minutes a day doing a short meditation where you switch off, relax and spend a few minutes picturing the detail of your vision without any distractions. There are many guided meditations out there to help you do this. I used to find them for free on YouTube, or download meditation apps. You may be practised enough to create your own meditation that allows you to switch off and see images of your vision without any guidance, and that's great. For me, guided meditation provided a structure to follow that helped me get in the zone more easily than if I did it myself. See what works for you. It could be that you need to try a few out to find one that works for you. When you're doing this, consider small things, like finding a voice that works for you, as well as the right tone and language. I still do this now with new goals in my life. Try out a few to find a style that works for you. If nothing else, it will build a bit more relaxation into your day, which is always good for your health and hormones.

CHAPTER 15

MAKE SELF-CARE A PRIORITY

Creating a new routine isn't always easy at first, especially when you have a busy life, so self-care is critical to help you manage the ups and downs of this journey.

Trying to conceive can be filled with a rollercoaster of emotions. You start the month full of hope and excitement. Then, once you've ovulated, the doubt kicks in, only to be followed by disappointment when your period arrives. I'm not going to pretend that if you follow this training, you won't have bad days. That's not realistic – it's more than likely that you will experience some personal setbacks and disappointments along the way. It's okay to feel down when things go wrong and it's good to let those feelings out, rather than bottling them up. What's critical is how you deal with the bad days and how quickly you recover. You can use these tools to manage any triggers that may set off a mindset meltdown. You can also use them to reframe the setback in a more positive way that enables you to move on and bounce back more quickly, avoiding disrupting your long-term plan.

Looking after yourself is critical in this process, and therefore self-care is another essential ingredient in your mindset tools. Very often we worry about everyone else, putting ourselves last. Or we distract ourselves by being so busy that we get burnt out and don't have time to do the things that make us really happy. We can also feel guilty about taking time out for ourselves! It may feel like a luxury we shouldn't be indulging in, but we have to remember how important it is to look after ourselves, especially when we are trying to conceive.

I'd like you to commit to self-care as you go through this process. Make yourself a priority every day, which means making time for your mindset training and looking after yourself – physically and mentally. Self-care is about having time just for you, to do the things that make you feel good and restore your energy.

Top tips for self-care

1. BE YOUR OWN BEST FRIEND

One critical tool to learn is how you talk to yourself when things go wrong. On this fertility journey, you are dealing with one of the toughest, most emotional situations you will face in life, and yet your mind can destroy your confidence and self-belief even further through negative self-talk. I often frame it as the best-friend scenario. If your best friend was in the situation you are now, would you be saying to them, "It's never going to happen to you. You don't deserve this. Everyone else will get pregnant except you"? Of course you wouldn't! So why do you talk to yourself like that? You need to change this hideous soundtrack in your head, and instead of being your biggest critic, become your biggest supporter, talking to yourself in a compassionate, caring way, instead of destroying your confidence on a daily basis.

2. RESPOND COMPASSIONATELY TO YOUR TRIGGERS

As you go through this journey, there will always be triggers, which are the experiences around us that instantly set off a mindset meltdown. This could be a friend telling you they are pregnant, seeing a pregnant woman at the supermarket or going to a social event filled with families. You may be practising all the positive tools in this book religiously, but if you are faced with a trigger unexpectedly, it can be too much to cope with, and before you know it, you are spiralling down the mental black hole again.

What doesn't help in this scenario is the negative self-talk you immediately revert to. You might start thinking things like, "I don't deserve a baby," or, "I will never get there." These thoughts are completely unhelpful! Remind yourself that you would not speak to your best friend in this way, so why are you doing it to yourself? Try to identify a more compassionate response instead, one that is more comforting. It could be something like, "Don't worry, your time will come," or, "You will get there," or, "You are next, you deserve this." Another way to respond compassionately is to remind yourself of your personal affirmation. Whatever words you use, your response doesn't have to hold all the answers – it just needs to be respectful, comforting and supportive.

3. CREATE A BANK OF MOOD SHIFTERS

We know that negative thoughts create bad feelings that keep our energy levels low and stop us from taking the action we want.

If you are having a bad day or feeling low, it's not always easy to "think" yourself out of that situation, like you might do on the good days. Instead, you may need to take deliberate steps to change your state of mind and shift your mood. You know what it's like – you have those days where you have been invited out and you just don't feel like it. You might force yourself to go and then you end up having a great time. Something happened there to shift your mood, whether it was having a good laugh with your friends, or perhaps talking about something other than getting pregnant. Whatever you did was a distraction and forced you to relax a bit more and enjoy the present moment, instead of dwelling on what's wrong in your life.

You can create a list of your own mood shifters that work for you. These are things you can do that will purposefully shift you to a better mood. These are some that work for me, but you can create your own list.

Music – Music is a huge passion of mine, and blasting out a favourite song is always guaranteed to change my mood for the better.

Movement – There is evidence to show that exercise releases endorphins, the feel-good hormones. This could be something active, like going for a run or hitting the gym, or a gentler exercise, like walking, yoga or even just dancing around your kitchen. Whatever you choose to do will have a positive impact on your mood. You may not feel like it beforehand, but force yourself to do some kind of movement and notice how it makes you feel afterwards. Remind yourself that it's unlikely you will ever regret doing some exercise, but you may regret not doing it!

Comedy – Laughter is a proven medicine. When was the last time you belly-laughed? Or laughed so much you had tears in your eyes? Put on a movie that is guaranteed to make you laugh, listen to a funny podcast while you are making dinner or arrange a night out with friends you know you have fun with.

Nature – Get out into nature and appreciate the beauty around you. This will help you to be more mindful and grateful, and will create a shift in your mood.

Time to yourself – Life is busy. We cram so much into our days, and we don't stop. When was the last time you did something just for you? It's important to look after yourself and keep your self-care bank topped up, especially when you are having a tough time emotionally. Do something just for you, whether that's a hot bath, massage, walk, trip to the cinema or even just time to read a book in the garden. It may feel indulgent, but you are definitely worth it, and it's a great mood shifter.

Practise being mindful – When you've been trying to conceive for a while, your head can become consumed with worry and anxiety about whether or not you will ever get pregnant. This means your mind is not often in the present moment. Instead, it is focused on an unwanted future that may not even happen, and that creates feelings of anxiety in your life right now.

As you read in Chapter 9, one of the keys to leading a happier life is to be more mindful and keep your attention focused on what is happening in your life in the present, instead of an imagined, unwanted event in the future.

You can practise being mindful at any time of the day. By focusing on what you are doing right now, you can calm down your internal chatter and focus your mind on the present moment. How often do you have your morning coffee whilst scrolling through your phone? How about eating your lunch whilst on the go, or even going for a jog and running through your to-do list in your head? Multi-tasking is a great skill but it's not good for mindfulness!

Not all of these thoughts may cause you anxiety, but it's still good to practise mindfulness when you can. Try carving out some time in your day to deliberately give your mind a break from the incessant chatter and just "be". And turn your phone off for a while. It may feel overindulgent to do this when life is so busy and there is so much to cram into your day, but anything that makes you feel better is definitely worth the investment.

See if you can find just five or ten minutes a day when you can be more mindful. It could be when you are eating your breakfast, having your coffee, going for a run or walk, or taking a shower. Focus on the experience of the activity and switch your thoughts off for a few minutes.

4. JOURNALING

As you start practising these tools, you will automatically become more aware of what is going on in your head and how you talk to yourself. Journaling is a great way to reflect on your progress and see how far you've come. And writing things down will help you identify where there are patterns in your thinking and behaviour.

You may be making fantastic progress overall, but there will always be certain situations or events that trigger those old patterns of thinking. That's okay, you are a work in progress, and the key to self-improvement is being self-aware. If you are able to notice when these old patterns kick in, that's excellent! By taking a step back and noticing how you are talking to yourself, you will realize that these statements aren't necessarily facts – they are just repeated thoughts that your brain has created, and that means they can be changed.

Start recording your thought patterns, noticing what you are telling yourself, bad and good, and how it makes you feel. Record it on your phone if you're out and about because you will soon forget.

Also make a note of your progress on all your mindset work and anything significant that impacted it during your day. If you have time to do this every day, great, but if not, a few times a week is a brilliant start. Keep a mindset journal – what have you been grateful for that day, what were your trophy moments that you were proud of yourself for, and what do you notice that you still need to work on? This is a great way of looking back, seeing your progress and celebrating what's gone well.

5. CREATE YOUR OWN SUPPORT NETWORK

Trying to conceive can feel very lonely. I used to feel that no one truly understood what I was going through. I thought people felt so sorry for me, that they were worried about saying the wrong thing and, as a result, they would stop talking to me about having a baby at all. This meant I bottled it all up even more and my obsessive thinking got worse.

It's not always easy to talk to your partner either. They are in the same situation as you, but they can experience it all very differently. Some partners are very practical and like to try fixing things, which can be difficult when nothing can actually be fixed and all you want to do is have a good cry. I used to find that my partner would bounce back a lot quicker than me after disappointments and would be less emotional about it all. And some of my clients would moan that their partners could be quite flippant, saying things like, "Oh well, we can just try again," after a failed treatment, and after a miscarriage, "Well, we almost got there, let's just do it again!" One client said that their partner stopped talking about it altogether, as they were terrified of upsetting them.

These are all well-meaning responses from partners who are desperate to do the right thing, but they are not always the most helpful. The differences in how couples deal individually with their fertility journey can lead to feelings of not being understood, and this can create distance, meaning that before too long, communication can start to break down. Here are a few ways to build your support network, with your partner and beyond.

Keep talking – It's important to keep the communication flowing with your partner. Explain to them what you need from them emotionally and let them know that sometimes it's just about being listened to and empathized with, rather than them feeling as though they have to fix things. Your partner is not a mind reader, and sometimes in relationships you have to be quite direct to explain what you need from them. You may be worried about doing this, but in my experience, and particularly in my experience with men, I have found that often they are grateful to know what's expected of them! At the end of the day, I promise you they just want you to be happy, and believe me, it is crushing for them watching you go through this and feeling so helpless.

Find your supporters – Who are your biggest supporters in life? You know that friend who always has your back, doesn't judge you and just really cares about you? In the same way as with your partner, they may find it difficult to know how to support you going through this. Despite this, I have no doubt that they desperately want to be there for you. As I have been writing this book, a few of my friends asked if there would be a chapter on how to support people going through infertility, and so I have added that to my survival guides at the end.

This shows me that people do care – they really do – and that good friends are desperate to give you the right support on this journey.

Don't be afraid of reaching out to friends or family when you're having a bad day. In the same way as with your partner, let them know what you need from them. It could be that you just want to offload and you don't need them to fix things. Perhaps you could have a ten-minute phone chat, a quick cup of tea or an outing somewhere together. If you are able to unburden yourself and get things out of your head, you will release some of the stress and emotion of the situation, which is always good news for your hormones. Be brave and reach out when you feel low – I'm sure you will be pleasantly surprised at the support you receive back.

Search for online support networks – If you don't have those good friends, you could turn to one of the many support networks out there. There are numerous online communities filled with people who are trying to conceive and all going through the same journey together. They provide a fantastic opportunity to share experiences and emotions instantly, with people who completely understand what you're going through. They can be a huge source of support if you don't feel like you have anyone else to turn to. A word of caution though: my own experience with these communities was that they could become quite draining after a while. Although it was lovely to interact with those going through the same thing, I found that the stories of failure, failure and more failure were quite negative. I wanted to hear success stories to help keep me positive and lifted. Sometimes it was just too much to be surrounded by people who continued to be unsuccessful, even after years of trying. Even just the way I had to complete my profile on some of the sites was quite negative to see. I would log on and immediately be greeted with a long list of women with profiles reading something like this:

Sarah
TTC 12 years
3 ABs
5 IVFs
2 IUls

In this case, Sarah had been trying to conceive for 12 years, had 3 angel babies (AB was either a miscarriage or a still born) and tried various fertility treatments. And there were hundreds of profiles just like this. Some people had been on there for years and seemed to have formed really close relationships. It was almost as though these communities and their challenges were defining them. For me, I found it hard to focus on my positive vision of the future and the life I wanted when I was surrounded by all those stories of disappointment and grief. The participants were lovely and so supportive to each other, but the groups ended up having the opposite effect on me. Thinking back to the tools I learnt and the concept of what you think about comes about, I didn't want to hear about unsuccessful attempts all day long. But if you're someone who doesn't have a strong network of your own, you may find it helpful. Or you could dip in and out as you need to, so you are not overloading yourself. This is often what I did, logging on when I needed specific support rather than letting it consume my time every day.

Try counselling – The other option for support could be to have some counselling sessions, specifically the type of counselling that allows you to offload your thoughts and emotions. If you are struggling to bounce back after a disappointment and you are finding it difficult to talk to anyone about it, even your partner, I would suggest you consider some counselling. The sessions will provide time just for you, away from the distractions of your life, in a safe and confidential environment. Unlike with your friends, where the conversation can shift from topic to topic quite quickly, the counsellor will structure the session to focus completely on you and your needs. They will listen, be empathetic and help you manage the emotions of your situation.

Many fertility clinics offer counselling for free after a failed attempt at pregnancy. If this is offered, my personal view is that you would benefit from taking up the offer. All support is good, and counselling can provide a vital outlet for your feelings and emotions in a way that is different from talking to friends or family. Alternatively, you can find a good counsellor in your local network or gain a recommendation from your doctor. There are many counselling websites that provide recommendations.

6. ACUPUNCTURE

As we have talked about in this book, so much of the process of getting pregnant is out of your control, which can be hugely frustrating. But there are holistic treatments out there that may improve your chances of success and might be something to try as part of your self-care routine. When I was on my journey, I was always looking into the latest fertility-enhancing treatments. You name it, I tried it. Some I really enjoyed, and they felt quite indulgent, such as reflexology – a wonderful foot treatment that stimulates pressure points in the body. Others were slightly less pleasant, such as the Chinese herb drinks that I used to boil up twice a day and force myself to drink while holding my nose – absolutely hideous, and I paid for the pleasure too.

But one treatment I kept coming back to was acupuncture. This is a traditional Chinese medical treatment where fine needles are inserted at certain points of the body to balance the flow of energy and relieve health conditions and symptoms. I hadn't really come across acupuncture before I got to the IVF stage of my journey. At that time, there was emerging evidence that acupuncture may help the chances of IVF success. I used two different practitioners on two different rounds of IVF. The second one was the one that worked. Did acupuncture help the outcome? I have no idea, but the IVF worked, and that was all that mattered.

CHAPTER 16

COMMIT TO A REGULAR ACTION PLAN

Once you can start to move your mindset into the right place, that's where the next critical step kicks in – your action plan! It's easy to sit and dream about your baby coming along, but the reality is that we have to go out there and take tangible steps to make it happen. Having a plan of action will help you stay focused and moving forward, which in turn helps keep that mindset positive!

If you fail to plan, you plan to fail!

As with any goal in life, the action you take to move toward it is fundamental to your success. You can dream about having a new job, a new house or a new partner, but if you don't take the necessary steps, this will just end up being a pipe dream and never reality. The same goes for your fertility journey. After years of trying, it's easy to feel too overwhelmed to take any positive steps forward, and you may feel quite negative or cynical about trying something new. Instead, you find yourself drifting along without much happening, and the months or even years ticking by with no baby.

Studies show that the most successful people in life take regular and consistent action, even when they don't feel like it. A lot of people (myself included) show great enthusiasm at the start of a project and then lose interest a few weeks later, especially if things aren't going the way they want! It's the same with your fertility journey. It's easy to feel less motivated if you have been trying for a while – I know I did. Once I hit the black hole of despair, I was too consumed with "why me" to even consider doing anything differently. I became closed down to new ideas and if I did try something new, it was out of desperation, and deep down I was cynical about its success before I even started.

You may be thinking, "How can I plan anything when getting pregnant is completely out of my control?" Well, of course, the actual act of the sperm and egg successfully fertilizing might be in the hands of the gods, but there is so much else that happens before that critical point that you ARE in control of. For example, you have control over your mindset every day, your behaviour, how you look after yourself, the medical interventions you choose, the holistic support you choose, your life around you, your support network and, of course, how much stress you put on yourself. All of these things *are* within your control, and they all contribute in some way toward you getting pregnant.

I have come to realize that I am always better with a plan, in any area of my life. A plan keeps me focused, it gives me steps to follow to start making real progress, and it makes me feel completely in control. How about you? You know you want to get pregnant, but do you have a plan to get you there?

Exercise: Your pregnancy goals

Obviously, you want to be pregnant, we know that! Getting pregnant is your overarching long-term goal, but if you have been trying to conceive for three years, then having a goal of "getting pregnant" may seem huge and totally beyond your reach. As a result, this goal ends up having the opposite effect and can be completely overwhelming, meaning that you have no idea where to start and what new steps to take. Instead, you bury your head in the sand, do nothing and end up drifting along with nothing changing.

What's important is to set some shorter-term goals to give you practical steps that you can follow right now. This puts you firmly back in control of your fertility journey, and you can immediately start to take small, positive steps toward your goal of getting pregnant.

Consider your timelines

Think about your timelines for getting pregnant. When do you want to be pregnant by, realistically? You might be thinking, "Well, next month, obviously!" But that is a very short-term goal – it puts all your eggs in one basket and creates immense pressure for you. The odds of you getting pregnant next month are so much lower than getting pregnant at some point over the next 6 months or 12 months. With that extra time you've allowed yourself, you have so many more chances, and suddenly your goal will feel much more achievable.

When I've had clients going into IVF, I often talk to them about how many IVFs they are prepared to do. Quite often they are pinning all their hopes on the first go, and this creates so much pressure mentally. The chances of success over the course of three IVFs is significantly higher than doing just one, and thinking more long term will definitely take the pressure off.

When you think about your own goal of getting pregnant, I'd like you to think this way. Create a time period for when you want to be pregnant that feels realistic and achievable. You may want to change the focus to help make it more long term. For example, instead of being pregnant by a certain date, do you have a future event or time in mind where you would like to be a mum? Make a note of this below, along with your timescales.

MY PREGNANCY GOAL	MY TIMELINES

What are the steps to get you there?

Write your goal and timeline for becoming pregnant in the middle of a blank piece of paper, and then start thinking of all the different steps you need to take to get there. Write them around the goal, a bit like a mind map. What are the key steps you need to take to achieve your goal of getting pregnant?

If you're not sure what to put, here are some suggestions. Perhaps you need to start looking after yourself. You might want to eat more healthily, start taking some vitamins, drink more water. Maybe you need to get some medical tests done or start looking for a specialist or a fertility consultant. Perhaps you want to save up some money for treatment, or maybe you want to work on your mindset, to feel more relaxed and less stressed about your journey. There could also be some things you want to do in life before you get pregnant. You might want to have a holiday abroad, move jobs or buy a new house before you get pregnant. You might even have an issue in your relationship that you need to resolve before you get pregnant. Whatever your situation, there will be critical steps to take toward your goal of getting pregnant. Write down whatever comes to mind, a bit like a brainstorm.

MY PREGNANCY GOAL AND TIMELINE

THE STEPS I NEED TO TAKE TO GET THERE

Exercise: Your three-week action plan

I have found that three weeks is a good period of time for an action plan. It is long enough to make real progress but not so long that you lose motivation. Look at all the steps you wrote down on your mind map and identify the biggest priorities. Which of these steps will have the most significant impact on your journey to get pregnant? You may pick one or two things depending on how big they are.

Write each step as a goal for the next three weeks – what do you want to achieve? Make sure the goal is positive. For example, if you want to lose half a stone before you get pregnant, write this goal more positively: "I want to be ten stone."

The next step is to identify what you are going to do in the next three weeks to move yourself closer to this goal. Be detailed and specific with what you are going to do and give yourself some deadlines. The aim is to break down this goal into manageable, practical steps.

For example, if your goal is to find a fertility consultant, your action plan might look like this:

1. Speak to Kate's friend about her consultant for recommendation – by end of Thursday
2. Research online consultants in the area – before the weekend
3. Contact three clinics to find out costs and wait times – by end of next week
4. Book an appointment – three weeks

Check your commitment

How committed do you feel to cracking on with your action plan right now? Score yourself on a scale of 1–10, with 1 being

"I'm not motivated to do this at all," and 10 being "I am fully committed and ready to go." If you have a lower score, ask yourself what is stopping you from scoring higher. Quite often, a low score will hint toward some negative thinking that could be holding you back. Or it could be that this isn't the right first step for you to take after all.

Listen to the voice in your head and what it's telling you, even if it's negative or cynical. It will give you clues as to what is holding you back. If it is mindset related, you can use the mindset tools to create a new positive affirmation to replace the negative one you are hearing. If it's related to the action you're doing, try to work out what's behind the negative thinking. It may be that the focus for your action plan isn't right. Is there something else you should be doing first? Be really honest with yourself at this stage – it's okay to tweak and change things.

Even if you are scoring 8 or 9, ask yourself why it's not 10. There could still be something else there that is holding you back.

I had one client who was saying all the right things, but her motivation was still very low, and she wasn't taking the action she committed to in our sessions. After some discussion, it turned out that there were underlying issues in her relationship that, deep down, were making her anxious about getting pregnant, even though this was what she desperately wanted long term. As a result, this was stopping her from committing to her fertility action plan and when we realized this, it was a real light-bulb moment for her. As a result, we changed the focus of her action plan to be all about fixing the relationship issues first, and this worked much better.

Listen to those tiny voices inside your head that are not working with you on your action plan. Write down in your journal what you're noticing. The voice may be small, but it can still have a big effect on your mindset and your motivation to move forward.

Create some accountability

Research shows that people will take action when they are fully motivated and inspired, when they have an incentive (for example, being paid), or when they are accountable to someone. Think about your own levels of motivation. What will help inspire you to take action on your plan? Hopefully this goal of getting pregnant is so important to you that you will do what you need to do, but if that's not the case, think about what else you can do to create some accountability.

For example, you could share your action plan with your partner or your best friend and ask them to have a weekly follow-up with you. Or you could give yourself a reward or incentive for when you have completed it. How will you make yourself more accountable?

Your mindset routine

You've already committed to working on your mindset daily, and this routine needs to become part of your action plan. Now you have the tools, you can commit to a three-week period to practise them, alongside your practical action plan. Twenty-one days is the perfect time period to create new positive habits. What are you going to commit to doing on a daily basis for the next three weeks, and how will you build these activities into your day?

Example action plan

Overall pregnancy goal:	
To be pregnant by Mum's 70th birthday in 12 months	

Three-week goal / milestone:	Today's date:
Investigate options for next medical steps	5 June

Action plan to get there:	Deadline:
• Research local fertility clinics online including success rates and methods	End of the weekend
• Ask Zoe and Caroline which clinics they used and get their views	Thursday this week
• Book doctor's appointment for referral to a specialist or the clinic	Book appointment for anytime next week
• Research test and treatment options online so I understand them all before seeing anyone	Before Doctor's appointment
• Go back on pregnancy vitamins and take one every day	Daily

Mindset routine:	Progress:
Affirmation: I am perfectly healthy and ready to conceive • Repeat this affirmation any time I am on my own and first thing in bed • Write Post-it notes, put on bathroom mirror • Find a quote image with perfect heath and make that my phone screensaver • Change my password to perfecthealth-37 **Gratitude:** • Record gratitude every morning while I'm having coffee • Make an effort to thank partner for doing things for me • Look for things to be grateful for during my day • Identify one good thing about the day before bed if I have a bad day	

Vision: Summer's picnic with me and my husband, sitting on a picnic rug with a baby, sunshine, happy... local park • Set up a screen saver for the laptop with a photo of the park • Daily meditation on the vision • Find a family picnic image that fits with image – stick it on the bedroom mirror **Self-care:** • Do some exercise by myself three times a week – walk or run • Date night after payday • Talk to Claire (friend) about everything I'm doing and ask her to support me • Start journaling before bed to make a record of what I notice about my mindset – any trophy moments or dips	
Commitment level and accountability: 8 / 10 – weekly review with partner Sunday morning	

This is just an example to get you started. You can create your own action plan that works for you. It's good to write it down because it helps get you focused, increases your commitment and accountability, and you can monitor your progress against it over the three weeks. My main tip here would be to *keep it simple!* Don't overload yourself with too many actions that you won't stick to. Remember that lots of small changes add up to make major change. Create a simple action plan that works for you and is easy to stick to. Start small and you can always add to it later. Make a note of your progress and any observations in your journal as you go through the action plan – what's gone well and what has been more difficult for you?

At the end of the three weeks, you can repeat the process again with a new goal and action plan. I have often found that things change for people over a few weeks. Their journey may take a new twist or turn, and therefore the next three-week goal may be different to the last one. This is all absolutely fine and part of the journey. Be open to new ideas and new opportunities when they present themselves – they might just take you where you need to go.

What is ultimately important with your action plan, however it looks, is that you are moving forward and taking the steps you need to. If this isn't happening, ask yourself: why not? There may be clues in your commitment level. Is your goal the right goal? Is there something else going on that is affecting your motivation, or an issue with your mindset that you need to tackle first? Perhaps you have simply not given it enough time and you are giving up too early?

Remember that in carving out a new mindset routine, finding one that works for you and one that fits into your life can be trial and error. But stick with it and tweak it as you need to. Remind yourself that change doesn't happen overnight and, a bit like that flight path I mentioned, making just one small degree of change today can make a huge difference to where you end up further down the line.

MY THREE-WEEK ACTION PLAN

CHAPTER 17

YOU'RE READY TO GO!

We've covered a lot in this section. You've done a huge amount of self-analysis and you've learnt the tools that will start to shift your thinking. You've carved out a routine to build these new mindset tools into your daily life, and you're well and truly committed to getting started!

Alongside all this, you will have written your fertility action plan and worked out the next critical steps that will move you closer to your goal of getting pregnant. You have made fantastic progress – well done! You have already taken some very positive steps forward and you should be proud of yourself for taking time out of your busy life to work on YOU.

Next, it's all about putting what you've learnt into practice and committing to the next three weeks. Follow your daily routine and practise using the tools with any challenges you face along with the way. Start to notice how your life changes, however small that change may be. Move forward with your fertility action plan and record your progress and observations in your journal.

It may not all be plain sailing. We have spoken about the good days and the bad days on this journey, along with the disappointments and setbacks. But now you have the tools to help you cope with these and recover from them more quickly – you may even stop them from happening in the first place. If you miss a day, don't beat yourself up; just get back on track with everything the next day. Consistency is key, so keep going – it's only three weeks at a time, so just focus on that time period instead of looking too far ahead.

If you feel your motivation wavering, look at the bigger picture. Remind yourself that what you were doing before wasn't working, and that learning to manage your mindset is something you have full control over. You just need to invest some time and commitment to make it happen. The benefits in all areas of your life are huge. And of course, remember why you're doing all of this, and how much you want that baby. Focus on your vision of success wherever you can.

Record how you're feeling in your journal, along with the changes you start to notice. You could see changes in your life overall, or changes in how you're feeling. But there will be changes, just you see. I wish you every success and I am right behind you – I know you can do it!

PART FOUR

SURVIVAL GUIDES

Ten years is a long time to spend trying to get pregnant. Over that time, I faced many different challenges and obstacles, and I learnt a lot. I had to cope with most of my friends getting pregnant, I attended numerous social events with families, and I was regularly quizzed about when I was going to have a baby. On top of that, I faced a host of medical challenges and had to juggle those with a demanding job.

These guides share my insights into how to cope with some of the toughest parts of your fertility journey. They are a reference guide and source of support from someone who has been there and gets it.

CHAPTER 18

THE BABY SHOWER

It's the moment you've been dreading. The pastel-coloured invitation drops into your inbox and your heart sinks. Immediately, you go into panic mode, and that familiar cloud of depression sweeps over you. It doesn't feel that long since you got over the news of the pregnancy, but now you have to spend at least two hours talking about the baby, admiring the bump and cooing over the gifts. For everyone else, this is a fun and happy occasion, but for you it is torture, a painful reminder that you are not pregnant and you may never be part of this exclusive mummy club.

Next, the anxiety sets in. Should you go? Should you tell them you're sick and stay at home? Will you even be able to keep it together in front of everyone? The emotions are hugely conflicting. Of course, this is a good friend, and deep down you are so happy for them, but at the same time you can't help but feel a mixture of resentment, envy and anger that it isn't happening to you. On the one hand, you want to go and support your friend, but on the other hand, the thought of wearing the happy mask all afternoon whilst crying inside is too much to bear.

How do you manage these events whilst protecting yourself from more hurt at the same time?

Decide whether or not you're going to go. This will usually depend on how well you know the person. If they are in your close circle of friends, then your absence may be highly visible and may damage your relationship. At the same time, though, a close friend will most likely know what you're going through and will empathize with your worries about the event. They should understand if you feel you can't stay the whole time, if you leave before a certain point in the proceedings or if you ultimately feel it's too much and can't go.

If the baby shower is not for a close friend, perhaps a work colleague or someone you don't see regularly, you could simply consider not going. Your absence won't be especially noted, and most likely the people attending won't be aware of what you're going through. Thank them for the invite but make your excuses. Remind yourself that it is perfectly okay not to attend and that you are the priority. Sometimes the best thing to do is to put yourself first, remembering that self-care is at the top of your list while you're on this journey.

Consider the timing of the event. If you are in the middle of a fertility treatment, or have recently suffered a setback on your journey, then going to a baby shower may not be the best thing to do for your stress and anxiety levels. If you are in between treatments, or at a point where there is no immediate activity happening, then you might feel happier about going. Remind yourself that you are not superhuman and you need to do what is best for you at that time. The event might trigger a mindset meltdown and that's okay, but if you are in the middle of a medical cycle or a treatment it might be better to say no. You have a lot invested in this cycle – physically, emotionally and probably financially – and you want to give yourself the best possible chance of success. That means prioritizing your mindset and doing everything possible to keep positive. It's absolutely fine to say thanks but no thanks!

Enlist some support. If it's a good friend's baby shower, it's likely that you will have some other close friends there. Chat to one of them beforehand to explain your worries and ask if they can be your ally for the day. They can help you out with any awkward questions or rescue you if anything becomes too much. If there's no one like that at the event, then identify someone who can be on the other end of the phone for you, a person you can message or call in a quiet place who will send you a supportive word back.

Have an excuse ready. You may not want to stay the distance at the baby shower and that is totally fine. You could pre-empt this with the host by telling them upfront that you can only stay an hour or so. Have an excuse ready so that you can leave when the time is right for you. It may feel like you stand out like a sore thumb, but I promise you all the focus will be on the pregnant mum. There will be so much going on that your departure will be forgotten in a few minutes.

Prepare your responses to those awkward baby questions. Have a few stock answers ready so that you aren't triggered to get upset and instead know what to say. Quickly move the subject on to another topic. Focus on the other person and remember that people love talking about themselves! See my separate guide to dealing with intrusive questions to help you plan what to say.

Reward yourself afterwards. You went, you got through it, and you survived! This is a huge achievement, so give yourself a big pat on the back. Reward this trophy moment with some self-care, by doing something that will make you feel good. It could be a massage, a relaxing bath or an outing with your partner. If you do feel upset or depressed afterwards, that's okay. Allow those feelings to come to the surface rather than pushing them away. If you need a good cry, let it all out. Then use the mindset tools to get back on track when you're ready. Practise some gratitude, remind yourself about what is good in your life now and that your time will come at the perfect moment for you.

CHAPTER 19

DEALING WITH INTRUSIVE QUESTIONS

When I think back on my own journey to pregnancy, I distinctly remember all the questions. When people know you are newly married or planning a life together, they just expect the little ones to come along, and they feel they have every right to ask about it! Here are some of the most common intrusive questions – and how you can reply:

"Are you planning to have children?" This is the big one. Quite often it pops out in small talk. Once you've got married or moved in together, this is the next obvious step. When this question comes up, it's important to decide from the outset how much you are prepared to share.

A simple answer that tends to shut things down is, "Not yet." There isn't much more people can say to that, is there? Or, if you want to be a bit more open, you could say, "Hopefully soon!" Sometimes being vague like this can be better than shutting the conversation down entirely. If you reply with something like, "I'd rather not talk about it, thanks," you could end up causing more intrigue, resulting in more questions from the other person.

If you decide to be more honest and say, for example, that you've been trying and it hasn't happened yet, you must be prepared for the questions that follow. Choose who you want to have this kind of conversation with carefully. Pick someone you can trust to confide in and don't be afraid to ask them to keep it to themselves – people love to gossip!

"Have you tried...?" When you start to explain that you have been trying to have a baby and it hasn't yet happened, you may find you have well-meaning friends who are keen to share their experience of what worked for them or the "miracle cures" they have heard about. They are full of tales of the neighbour's cleaner who swore by lying with their legs in the air for 20 minutes after having sex, or the woman in the local shop who took aspirin to help the embryo embed into the womb. Or better still, their colleague at work who decided to "just relax and forget about it", only to find out they were pregnant the next month!

You may feel like steam is coming out of your ears when you hear these stories. These people have no idea about the depth of your struggle and how you have tried absolutely everything under the sun, including relaxing (although we know that's not always an easy one!). Take a deep breath, listen and be patient! Remind yourself how much they care about you and that they are just trying to help. Acknowledge what they're saying with comments like, "That sounds interesting." Better still, thank them for trying to help. Or you could decide to share more about your journey with them. By opening up and telling them exactly what you have been going through, they may have a better understanding of just how heartbreaking this situation is for you, and how much you have tried already.

"How is the IVF going?" You may have got to the point that you are having fertility treatment and have told a few people in your circle this is happening. Fast-forward to the next social gathering, and someone asks you how it is all going. There could be a few scenarios here. Perhaps you are happy to talk about it but not in the middle of a pub with lots of people about. Chances are, you may get emotional when you're talking about it and you don't want to cause any fuss. You could reply with something like, "Okay, thanks, but maybe we can talk about it another time on our own and not here." Or you could say, "It's going okay, thanks, but I'd rather not talk about it with everyone else around."

I sometimes used to say, "I can't really talk about it because I might cry," which ended up being completely the wrong thing to say because it prompted an outpouring of sympathy from the other person, which would then set me off anyway! Decide how much you want to share at more public gatherings and think about how you will respond to these questions.

"Do you know what's wrong with you? Whose fault is it?" This is a very personal question. When people don't have an emotional connection to the situation, they may see it as an obvious question to ask. They don't realize the sensitivity that comes with it. In this scenario, don't feel pressured into sharing too much. Even if you are comfortable talking about the medical reasons behind your fertility, your partner may not want you discussing their sperm quality in public!

Giving a vague reply can be helpful to shut the conversation down, for example, "There are a few minor things but we're working through them." Or, if you have a diagnosed condition, you may want to divulge what it is but without sharing too much, e.g., "Well, I've got endometriosis, so our treatment is based on that." If your partner is the issue, consider using a vague response rather than divulging their personal information.

"With all the unwanted children out there, why don't you just adopt?" Lots of people are very happy to consider adoption without realizing what a difficult journey it can be, both emotionally and financially. Some people are lucky, but there can be lengthy processes in place with lots of red tape and detailed assessments that have to be carried out. Also, things have moved on from the '50s where women were giving up their babies if they weren't married. This means there are fewer babies and more children to adopt, who may have been in care for a few years. There is a lot for couples to consider before going down this route, and there can be many disappointments along the way. You hear stories of people getting to the final hurdle, including meeting their potential child, only to be disappointed at the last minute. It is almost as heartbreaking as not conceiving. Explain how difficult the process can be and what is involved emotionally and financially.

You may be concerned that you are being judged for not considering adoption. Once again, remind yourself that this is your journey and only you know the depths of what you have been through to have a child. Everyone has different ethics and values. Some people want to adopt from the start, others want to do everything they can to have their own child first. Either way is totally acceptable, and other people's opinions really don't matter.

CHAPTER 20

YOUR FRIEND IS PREGNANT

It's the news you have been dreading. A good friend has finally got pregnant and announces this to you when you meet up, completely out of the blue. What started out as quite a good day is immediately shot to pieces, and up pops the negative chatter in your mind: "It's not fair, why can't this happen to me? I will never be the one that gets pregnant." Of course, you are happy for your friend's news, but you can't help but feel sad as it's another reminder that it's not happening to you. So how do you handle this situation?

Put yourself in their shoes. We can become quite self-obsessed on the journey to conceive, very much wrapped up in the situation and feeling that our pain is worse than anyone else's. It can be easy to forget what's going on in other people's lives. Try shifting your thinking to consider it from your friend's point of view. They are pregnant and that is ultimately amazing news! They will not have to go through what you are going through – you wouldn't wish it on anyone. Or maybe they have and you're just not aware of it. They are a really good friend, and of course you are happy for them. Say congratulations, ask questions about the pregnancy and, for a few minutes, focus your attention purely on them, not yourself.

Allow yourself to be upset if you feel that way. Once the conversation is done, or you've gone home afterwards, remind yourself that it is okay to feel upset. Allow yourself a little cry or to feel a bit down. Let those feelings out rather than bottling them up. Perhaps phone your partner or a family member who understands your situation and have a moan. Having a bad day is okay, but use your mindset tools to bounce back quickly afterwards.

Remember: your friend will be nervous about telling you. One of my good friends had three babies in the time I was trying to conceive, and I will never forget the look of anxiety on her face when she told me about the third pregnancy. "But it should be you," she said, with so much genuine compassion. She knew what I had been going through and she was really worried this news would upset me. Remember that your close friends *do* get it and will be worried about sharing this type of news with you. If you know a friend is trying to conceive, you could always talk about how best to share any pregnancy news when it comes. Perhaps it might be easier to get a text so you can digest the news first before seeing them. Remind yourself that you can open up to your good friends and that they really don't want to do or say anything to upset you.

CHAPTER 21

JUGGLING IVF WITH WORK

You're finally starting your fertility treatment – hurrah! Now you're in the hands of the medics. You're excited, and also nervous. But overall, you're full of hope that your baby is finally on its way.

Then you get your treatment schedule, and your heart sinks when you look at the number of appointments over the coming weeks. Blood tests, scans, consultants – and all during working hours, of course.

Juggling fertility treatment with a busy job can be hugely stressful. It was one of the reasons I packed in my job after my fourth IVF had failed. Many clients tell me they feel so anxious thinking about how they will manage it. And all this stress is not good for your hormones.

Fertility treatment is such a private journey. You don't want everyone in the office knowing what you're doing. But at the same time, you need to take time off without worrying that disappearing every five minutes will set tongues wagging. And then there's the effect on your career. Will the boss think you're not committed anymore? Will you be passed over for that promotion?

Here are my top tips for juggling fertility treatment with a busy job:

Confide in your boss. It might not be a conversation you really want to have, but you'll be surprised at how supportive your boss might be if you open up. Getting time off (often at short notice) is likely to be much easier if they are in the loop. Be honest about how much time you will need and make an agreement upfront as to how to manage it. And consider what you will both say to the wider team. Doing this before the treatment starts will mean you go into the process feeling calmer and more in control, without the stress of worrying how to deal with unexpected appointments or questions from work.

Check your company's HR policies. How much time off are you entitled to? Most HR policies will allow people to take a reasonable amount of time off for hospital appointments, and some policies now even allow for IVF. You might need proof of your appointments. If you're not getting the right support from your boss, consider involving the HR team. They are there to make sure you are treated fairly and given the support you are entitled to.

Don't overload your day. Wherever possible, try to avoid making your day too stressful. Don't cram in too many meetings because you feel bad that you've got to leave at 2pm for a scan. Put yourself first. You've got a lot invested in this, financially and emotionally! It's only a few weeks and before you know it, normality will resume. Remember, it's all about keeping yourself calm and positive during the treatment process. Again, get support from your boss or HR to do this where needed.

Work out what time off you need. Depending on your job, you might find it easier to take some time off. You could take annual leave or ask your consultant to sign you off for a few days when you have busy appointments, or even after your treatment. My job was extremely busy, so it helped me physically and emotionally to take a few days off after the embryo transfer, to keep the stress levels down. However, everyone is different, and some people like to be distracted instead of putting their feet up all day. Just make sure you're not working too hard or creating any unnecessary stress. Your priority is to put yourself first and leave work on time!

Manage your mindset. Self-care is the priority during this treatment, and that starts with what's going on mentally.

If you're worried about how much time you're taking off and what everyone thinks you're doing, it will affect your stress levels. Remind yourself of why you're doing this and the importance of it all. Who cares what other people think?! They are not your concern, and you can't control what's going on in their heads. You are investing too much in this, both physically and emotionally, to give it anything other than 100% mentally. Focus on yourself, not what may or may not be going on around you. Things will be back to normal in a matter of weeks. Do whatever you can to stay positive during your treatment – use your affirmations, practise gratitude and visualize yourself with a positive outcome. You've got nothing to lose so give it EVERYTHING.

CHAPTER 22

MOTHER'S DAY

So, Mother's Day has come round again. Another reminder that everyone else has the baby you so desperately want. I always found this day tough, and it didn't help that the build-up to it seemed to last for weeks. It was impossible to escape the cards and gifts that were in my face everywhere I went.

One year, my lovely goddaughter sent me a Mother's Day card... a really nice gesture, I thought. It gave me faith that those close to me hadn't forgotten what I was going through, or how hard it was for me.

So here are my tips to coping with this annual event, without totally losing the plot:

Remember you are not alone. The brain always sees what we're looking for. Therefore, on Mother's Day you will see mums! But there are so many women out there who are just like you and struggling through the same journey of trying to conceive. There are also women who long to be pregnant but haven't met the right partner yet. Or women who have sadly lost their mums, or even lost a child. Often on this journey it feels like we are the only one, but we're not.

Celebrate your own mum. Don't forget to appreciate the mother figure you have in your life. Once you have your own family, you won't have as much time to do this (believe me, you really won't!). It has been proven that being grateful increases happiness and decreases feelings of depression, which are both very important to the balance of your hormones when you are trying to get pregnant. So, do something nice with your mum, or one that you are close to.

Indulge yourself. Okay, you would prefer to be a mum, but how about spending the day doing the stuff you wouldn't have the luxury of doing as a mum? Have breakfast in bed, watch movies all day, book a massage, go to the theatre, go to the seaside – do whatever makes you happy. You will look back at those times so fondly when you do have your family, especially when the only time you get to yourself is in the toilet – and you think I'm joking!

I don't mean to be flippant when I say "*when* you become a mum", because how you talk to yourself internally is so important in achieving what you want. We want less of the "if" and more of the "when". Do you think Mo Farah ever said, "I'm just not sure if I will ever win the 1500 metres"? He knew damn well he would, and that's exactly what he did. Making subtle changes to the language you use internally will help to shift your mindset and keep you more positive about the future and your ability to get pregnant.

So, before you know it, another Mother's Day will be over, and hopefully next year you will be celebrating for different reasons. But in the meantime, make a fuss of yourself, and your own Mum... you both deserve it.

CHAPTER 23

FRUSTRATIONS WITH THE MEDICAL PROCESS

When we are on the journey to pregnancy, we find ourselves completely in the hands of the medics. They are the experts, of course, so we hang on their every word, we do what they tell us to do, and we have faith that they're putting us on the right path.

But what happens if somewhere down the line, we start to lose a bit of that faith? Maybe the process that we've been following isn't working, or we're hitting endless setbacks along the way. Perhaps the speed of the system is frustrating the hell out of us, or maybe the medics make a flippant negative comment that we just can't get out of our heads.

This can all start to affect our mindset, and how we feel about the path we're taking. Having doubt in our heads is not good if we want to get pregnant.

This happened to me around the time that I had done four IVFs, with one miscarriage along the way. At that point I hit rock bottom and lost the faith. The official advice was to "keep going – there's no reason why it won't work at some point", but deep down I just wasn't comfortable with that. For starters, the cash was seriously running out. But also, it just seemed crazy – doing the same thing over and over again and expecting a different result. After all, that's the definition of madness, isn't it? I knew something had to change, and hot off the back of my mindset shift, I decided I wasn't accepting it.

I sat down in front of my consultant, who was expecting me to book my next treatment, and I said I wasn't doing it again until I had more tests. I could see the frustration in his eyes as "officially" there was nothing wrong with me, but luckily, he was the nicest, calmest man, and he just asked me what kind of tests I wanted. *Err... I don't know, you're the expert!* I launched into my theory that there must be more they could carry out to find out why it wasn't working, that something had to be wrong, and quite often I felt like I was pregnant in the early stages but then all the feelings would disappear overnight. There had to be more tests they could do.

Eventually, he said I could have the miscarriage tests. These are the tests you get for free on the NHS in the UK after you've had three miscarriages, or you can pay for them privately at any time, but most people won't be aware they exist. I mean, seriously, it takes three baby losses before you can get tested?

We decided to pay for them, and they did come up with something: a slight chromosome abnormality that might have been a problem or might not have been. But as a result, they tweaked the drugs I was on. Mentally, that helped me believe I was doing something different and, combined with my new mindset tools and a bit of acupuncture, hey presto, it finally worked for me, and three times over with the triplet pregnancy!

Great news for us, I know, but my point is this: I knew deep down that the path we were on wasn't right. I knew something had to change and, luckily, I had the confidence and drive to push for it. If you have the same nagging feelings, consider these three things:

Don't be afraid to ask questions and challenge the advice you're given. Okay, you're not a medical expert but you are an expert as far as your own body is concerned. The goal of getting pregnant is the most important thing in your life right now, and you've got to be on a mission with it. If something doesn't feel right, change it. Don't leave any stone unturned or any questions unanswered.

Consider getting a second opinion. As far as fertility goes, there are lots of different views out there. If you're not happy with the medical opinion, the consultant or the clinic, go somewhere else. Don't let excuses like time and money get in your way. You might say things to yourself like, "But it will take too long to change clinics," or, "It's more expensive to see that consultant." Come on, how much do you really want this? You've got to be happy with the path you're on; otherwise, your mindset will be out of sync with what you're doing. You're investing a huge amount of time, money and emotional energy in this – don't continue with your treatment with any mental conflict.

Be open to new opportunities around you. Keeping an open mind is so important on this journey. There is a whole world of medical support out there – it doesn't just stop with your GP and local fertility consultant. Do your research, speak to people who have been successful, look into recommendations you are given and explore opportunities that pop up unexpectedly. It's easy to close down new ideas by judging them too quickly or making excuses not to consider them, especially if it's not on the more traditional route. Look into everything and research everything. Treat this goal of getting pregnant like any other goal in your life and be tenacious in considering every option that comes along!

Trust your instincts. Listen to what your inner voice is telling you. There's a difference between the negative, fearful chatter that can stop you achieving what you want, and the trusting, knowing gut instinct you get about things. Basically, if you feel any fear, it's probably the former. Learn to know the difference and listen to what your gut is telling you – it's usually right.

CHAPTER 24

SECONDARY INFERTILITY

When I started coaching other people on a fertility journey, I was amazed by how many of my clients were coping with secondary infertility. Isn't it strange how the body can produce one child perfectly easily and then grind to a stubborn halt for the next one? Often in these cases the infertility is unexplained, so there is the added frustration and shock that comes from falling pregnant very easily the first time round and then not being able to do it the next time.

What I noticed with these women was that their desperation and desire to get pregnant was just as strong as those without any children. They didn't feel complete without another child and the emotions they were experiencing were just as heartbreaking as those without any children.

Judgements

For these women I think there are a number of added pressures to their situation. For starters, there is the judgement from the people around them who just don't get it. How many times have you heard well-meaning friends or family members say, "Well at least you already have one child"? Well yes, you do have a child and you are eternally grateful for that. But why aren't you allowed to dream of a bigger family just like everyone else does? The people who make those comments most likely already have their own second or third child. So how can it be okay for them to want a second child and go on to have one, but you have to accept a limit on your family?

And with this judgement comes the guilt that you should be grateful for what you've got, and not be greedy by wanting more children. You may find that people judge you for continuing to put yourself through fertility treatment and spending thousands of pounds when you already have one healthy child. Surely one child is enough? Why on earth would you put yourself through this? But it's not enough, is it? The longing for that bigger family won't just go away.

I can remember a friend of mine having a miscarriage when she already had two older children, and the first thing that came out of my mouth was, "Well, at least you know you can get pregnant." Ouch! Not very supportive! But for these women, it all added to their feelings of being misunderstood and alone in the situation. With my clients, I often found that their partner wasn't as keen to keep trying for a second child, they were more often happy to have just one. This became another reason for those women to retreat inside themselves, isolate their thinking and, before they knew it, another mindset meltdown had arrived.

The child you already have

One of the toughest aspects of dealing with secondary fertility is the impact on the child you already have. One of my best friends said that, every year, her daughter would ask Father Christmas for a baby brother or sister. She would look at her with desperate eyes and say, "Why does everyone else have a baby brother or sister and not me?" As if getting pregnant wasn't hard enough without the small person you love most in the world begging you for a baby that you are unable to produce! And then there's the age gap. You know how it works. You imagined having two children, just a couple of years apart, who did everything together and became the best of friends when they were older. And of course, when you're out and about, it's those typical families that you see. But it hasn't worked out that way. Instead, you are faced with a much bigger age gap than you planned, perhaps even five years or more. You start to worry about the implications of having such a big gap – how on earth will it work? Once again, the brain chatter starts and the anxiety is off and running.

Quite often, your partner may not have the same desire for more children that you do. If they were really honest, they might say they are content with one child and they are only going along with the second pregnancy to keep you happy. This can put added pressure on your relationship at a time when you are already managing the parenting challenges of a baby or young child. This, in turn, can have a knock-on effect on your sex life, which is not good when you're trying for a baby.

So how do you manage this journey with all these challenges facing you?

Be accepting of the situation. Remind yourself that, in the end, everything happens just at the right time. If you have a five-year age gap between your children instead of the two-year gap on your preconceived timeline of life events, it's important to remind yourself that it's okay and it will work just as well. Look at the rest of your life and consider: where else have you planned to do something, only for it to work out differently in the end? Perhaps your relationships, your work successes or the life choices you have made? Did things work out exactly as you had planned? I would hazard a guess that they may not have. And it's highly likely that will be the same for when your second baby decides to come along. The sooner you can bring yourself to accept the situation and be open to a new timeline with a more flexible age gap between your children, the more relaxed you will be on this journey. And there are benefits to a bigger age gap… you will have a little helper, for starters!

Nurture your relationship. Do whatever you can to nurture your relationship through this challenging time. Talking about how you are both feeling is critical to keep you connected on this journey. If you are finding it difficult to talk about the situation, book some counselling together, or find a fertility coach. You could also ask your GP about specialist support groups for secondary infertility. When you talk to your partner, find out if you are both on the same page with it all. What can you do to support each other through this difficult time? Partners aren't always the best mind readers, and sometimes it can be helpful to tell them directly what kind of support you need.

Carve out small pockets of time you can spend with your partner to reconnect. With a young child to manage, this isn't always easy. It could be something simple, like not turning on the TV one night or having dinner together when the baby is sleeping. Or you could get someone to look after your child for a few hours so you can go for a walk or grab a bite to eat – time to connect and a bit of a break from being parents too. The routine of being parents is exhausting, so it's important that you look after your relationship and talk through your feelings, or just have some fun together away from home.

Consider your lifestyle. Take a good, hard look at your lifestyle right now. What has changed since you had the first baby? If you are busy being a new parent, chances are you will have less time to look after yourself. What are you doing differently since last time? If you got pregnant very quickly the first time, you may not fully understand how your lifestyle impacts your ability to conceive. Buy a good book that outlines all the basics and see how you match up. Are you remembering to eat healthily, take your vitamins and drink lots of water? I know when I had small children, my needs were often last on the list. Do you have more stress in your life now compared to the first time, and are you getting enough sleep? As we have talked about earlier in the book, the balance of hormones in your body is hugely delicate and can be easily affected. Remember to consider your partner too – are they drinking more coffee (or alcohol!) since the last pregnancy? Both of these things can have an impact on sperm count.

Try and be really honest with yourself about what is different this time round. Work out where you can (both) make some positive changes and remind yourself that your self-care is critical. As a new mum, this is often low on the list of priorities, so that is something that needs to change!

Check your health. How is your health? Do you have any new health issues since your first pregnancy, or any chronic conditions that may have got worse? Be objective and honest with yourself about this – it's easy to ignore symptoms or dismiss them as irrelevant. Go to your GP in the first instance and ask to be checked out for fertility. Your GP can do the basic checks and make a referral to a specialist if needed. If you don't want to wait, consider booking a private appointment at a female health clinic. And don't forget to check out sperm quality too. Any fertility specialist, whether you are paying privately or not, should be able to carry out a full assessment of your health and hormones. You need to know what's going on inside, and if you get a clean bill of health, that will help you feel more positive. But if anything does come up, it's good to be aware of it early so that you can get the necessary treatments in place.

Manage your mindset. In this book, I have described how the mindset can work against you on any kind of fertility journey. It's no different with secondary infertility. As time goes by, you may fall into the trap of subconsciously doubting that you will ever achieve your dream of a second child. I had one client who was about to go into fertility treatment, and at one of our first sessions, she said that they had already decided what they would do if it didn't work. As such, both her vision and her plan were based around the treatment not working! I totally understand how this happens and why we avoid thinking about what we truly want to try and protect ourselves from yet another disappointment. But it's so important for you to focus on the future you WANT, not the one you don't want.

Focus on family life. Coping with the emotions of any fertility struggle can be hard. Don't let the emotions of secondary infertility push you away from your partner and your child. As you have learnt in this book, focusing on anything that brings you joy in your life will help to keep you happy and your mind present, instead of feeling anxious about the lack of pregnancy. Children are a wonderfully innocent distraction, and it's critical that you make time to enjoy your family life and be grateful for what you have now. Remember that the universe loves grateful people!

Avoid worrying what others think. You can't control the comments that other people make about your secondary infertility, whether it's the judgements and the criticisms, or just the lack of understanding about why you want another baby so badly. It's important to accept that you can't influence other people's views no matter how you respond to them, and this will help you to let go of those comments and stop you feeling guilty. Remind yourself that this is YOUR journey and you have every right to want a second child, just as much as everyone else does. Most people in your situation would feel exactly the same way you do – and that includes the people with bigger families who just got lucky! So, when you hear these types of comments, remind yourself that their opinion is not important and let them go.

Make an action plan. Family life is busy, so it's important that you make time to create a plan to address your secondary infertility. When you have a baby or a toddler in tow, the days can fly by, often without achieving very much at all except getting through the day. And on a bad day, you may not even get dressed or manage to leave the house! This can make it harder to find the time to take steps forward. When you're busy with children, it can be easy to feel too overwhelmed or tired to do anything. Go back and read the section on action planning in Chapter 16 to help you create a plan for your fertility journey. Set yourself some goals, whether that's going to see a medical professional or simply making changes to your lifestyle. Remind yourself that drifting along and just hoping something will change will not achieve anything. You are the only one who can move things forward.

The other reason to take action is for the child you already have. If your child is constantly asking you when they are getting their baby brother or sister, just like all their friends, the pressure can be immense. You want to be able to look them in the eye and tell them that you are doing everything you possibly can to have another baby, whether that's medical steps or more practical lifestyle steps, and that starts with making time to create a plan.

CHAPTER 25

SUPPORTING A FRIEND ON A FERTILITY JOURNEY

When I started telling people I was writing this book, a lot of them asked if there would be anything about how to support someone going through the challenges of trying to conceive.

When someone has been on this journey a while, it can be easy for them to start withdrawing and avoid talking to friends and family about their situation. On the one hand, they might feel you don't understand what they're going through, and on the other hand, you aren't sure exactly how best to support them, particularly if you have never experienced infertility yourself.

As a result, the whole journey can become a taboo subject or, at worst, you don't know what to say so you end up saying nothing at all, and this only adds to their feelings of loneliness.

So how do you support a friend or family member on this journey?

Ask what support they need. This might seem obvious, but it's not always easy to do, especially if you are worried about upsetting them. Everyone is different, so the type of support that works for you may be different to what they need. They may be relieved you are asking them upfront, as people on this journey don't always find it easy to talk about what they're going through. They may not want to be a burden and, as such, by asking them, you are creating a safe environment for them to open up.

Offer practical support. It can be useful to offer specific practical support so that your friend knows you are there for them and you're thinking about them. Offer to go to appointments or scans with them, even if it's just to sit in the waiting room or hold their hand during any procedures. If they are doing an exercise or diet programme, offer to join them for part of it. Suggest a movie night or a café outing. Book a treat you know they would enjoy.

They may not always say yes, but by making these specific gestures of help, you are showing that you care and really are there for them when they need you. Believe me, it will absolutely be appreciated, and it will remind them that they are not on their own and they do have a support network around them.

Find out the basics of what they're going through. If they are about to embark on IVF, read up on it so you understand the process. If they have been diagnosed with endometriosis, research the condition on the internet. Having a bit of background info about what they are facing will create a more meaningful conversation when you next see them. You can ask more informed questions about the process and understand the steps they will be going through.

Ask how they are... and listen! Take time to ask your friend how they are doing. They may find it difficult to open up or to start a conversation about their situation, so doing this is a reminder that they do have people around them who care. Start the conversation using open questions such as:

- How are you?
- How is it all going with baby planning?
- How is the treatment going?
- What's the latest with the baby plans?
- How are you feeling about it all?
- Do you want to talk about it?

If they don't want to talk about it, they might say so, and that's fine – don't be offended, some people are more private. But don't assume that by not mentioning it themselves they don't want to talk about it – quite often they just don't know where to start.

Avoid trying to fix the problem. If you don't know how to respond when they start talking, just listen and empathize. When you don't know what to say, it's easy to feel like you need to fix the situation for them or offer a solution, but very often this isn't what they need at all. It's more likely they just want to be listened to, understood and empathized with. If you're not sure what to say, try one of these responses:

- "I'm so sorry to hear that."
- "I can hear how tough it's been for you."
- "That must have been really hard."
- "I'm really sorry you're going through all this."
- "I'm here to listen whenever you need me."
- "What can I do to help you?"

Avoid those well-meaning cliché responses. You know the ones I mean! They usually pop out when you are trying to say the right thing and desperately want to make the person feel better. Quite a lot of these responses start with the words "At least …"

- "At least you can try again."
- "At least you already have one baby."
- "At least you know you can get pregnant."
- "At least you've got each other."
- "At least you don't have the sleepless nights like I do."
- "At least you're fit and healthy."

Mmmm! These statements are usually said with the best intentions, but sadly they only minimize what the person is going through and imply they are somehow lucky to not have a baby when they really want one – not really what they want to hear at all! They don't need you to make them feel better, they just need you to LISTEN and empathize.

If you do say the wrong thing, that's okay – you're only human. Just be honest, quickly apologize and say you don't always know the best thing to say. And reassure them that you are there for them, to listen or provide other support, depending on what they need.

Be consistent with your support. Aim to show the person going through this journey that you are there to support them throughout the whole process. Try to do so by being as consistent as possible with your support. Arrange regular catch-ups and check in to see how they are doing by text or phone, rather than giving loads of support at the start and then trailing off.

Know that your support is appreciated. If you're reading this guide, you are clearly a person who wants to take the time and effort to provide the right support to someone on this journey. Believe me, that is most definitely appreciated. I was lucky enough to have a few of these people around me when I was going through it – people I knew I could turn to however I was feeling, whether I wanted to cry, laugh or get everything off my chest. Be confident that the support you are providing is making a big difference to their journey and they are very lucky to have you by their side.

CHAPTER 26

SOCIAL EVENTS WITH FAMILIES

My fertility journey started when I was 30 and finished when I was 40. For most of my best friends, this was the prime age for reproduction, and I seemed to be surrounded by people getting pregnant. Over those ten years, most of my best friends got pregnant, many twice and some three times. As a result, life was changing for all of us. Gone were the wild nights out, replaced with Saturday afternoons at the park and family barbeques in the summer, with children running around everywhere you looked.

I have always loved kids, and it was fantastic to play mum to some of my closest friends' children, but some days the pain of attending these events with lots of families was too much to bear. Here are my top tips for dealing with family social events:

It's okay to say no. On the good days, you can cope with being surrounded by children, but on the bad days, it's a lot harder to put yourself through it. Remember that sometimes it's okay to just say, "No, thank you," and not go. A good friend will understand and not get offended. Depending on who it is and your relationship with them, you can either be honest or, if it's easier, you can make up a harmless excuse. Remember that self-care is at the top of your list, and you will know the days when this is something you are able to cope with.

Reframe the situation. Looking back now, it's easy for me to see that I was looking at those happy families through rose-tinted glasses. I was seeing the smiles, the children laughing and playing, the parents proudly looking on, and I was desperate to have that life. I didn't know it at the time, but it was very likely that those smiling parents had only had a few hours' sleep the night before, or that the toddler had thrown a massive tantrum in the car before they arrived. Maybe they'd even had to take the week off work because both children had tummy bugs at the same time. I know now that parenting is tough and it's not all about kids skipping happily across a field of poppies. I wouldn't swap my life now for anything, but I do wish in hindsight that I had appreciated my calm, adult-only world a bit more when I had it! Try to keep a balanced view of what parenting is like and appreciate all the time you have to yourself right now, because once the baby comes along, that will all change forever.

Don't be too hard on yourself. These events are an in-your-face reminder of the life you want but don't have. You're only human and this is bound to upset you. I would go to these events with my happy mask on and pretend like everything was fine, which was exhausting and often left me completely drained. Don't beat yourself up if you feel down that night or the next day – that's okay. As we have learnt in this book, it's okay to have these moments, but what's important is that you use your mindset tools to bounce back quickly.

Don't stay too long. Decide in advance how long you want to stay for. An hour? Two hours tops? It may feel easier to cope with the situation at first, but then you could find yourself drained an hour later. Your early departure may feel conspicuous, but I promise you that everyone else is having too much fun to notice. If it makes you feel better, confide in the host and let them know in advance what you will be doing. Most people are understanding, and it avoids any questions on the day.

Practise your vision. This book is all about focusing on what you want rather than what you don't want. Look at these events differently. Think about them as an opportunity to practise parenting and help you hook into your vision of being a mum. I used to love playing mum with my godchildren at these events, and it was so special to create a close bond with them. I'm very lucky that my friends trusted me to take their children on little outings too, giving me the perfect opportunity to bring my vision to life. I loved every minute, and the memories are so special to look back on now.

CHAPTER 27

THE TWO-WEEK WAIT

Whether you're doing a formal fertility treatment, or just trying out a new medication or natural technique, there is no getting away from the dreaded two-week wait. It's that point in the monthly cycle where you have done everything you can do – you have ovulated, and your egg may have fertilized – and now you just have to WAIT to see whether you are pregnant.

For me, having done five IVFs and three IUIs, the two-week wait was always the longest two weeks of my life. Never have I counted down the days (and hours) so religiously. Never have the days and weeks dragged by so slowly, and never have I analysed every twinge and change in my body more than during that time.

So, what can you do to survive the two-week wait (or 2WW as it's commonly known) without going totally insane?

Keep busy, but don't overdo it. If you have done IVF, you will have already invested a lot into the past few weeks, both financially and physically with what your body has gone through. But don't blow all that good work now the embryos are back inside you. It's not the time to go back to your crazy, busy, stressful work routine. By all means, keep busy, but don't push yourself too hard. Don't do anything that is going to make you feel anxious or stressed, and avoid overloading your diary, especially with too much physical exertion. It's important to keep yourself calm and relaxed. Remember that the mental investment is as important as the physical and financial one – they are all pieces of the jigsaw.

Consider taking time off. Everyone is different, and you will know what works best for you in these two weeks. For me, I had a very busy, stressful job, so when I did IVF, I always took at least a week off work to let me relax, both physically and mentally. For me, just chilling at home was the perfect tonic when I was normally so busy. If you are similar, consider booking some annual leave, or ask your consultant to sign you off work during the treatment period. It's definitely worth considering if your work environment causes you any stress. Remind yourself how much you have invested in this treatment – physically, mentally and financially. You don't want to do anything at this late stage to jeopardize that investment, so carry on investing in yourself by taking the time off that you need.

On the other hand, I have had clients that would consider taking time off as their worst nightmare. They had no desire to sit around at home wondering whether or not they were pregnant. If this is you, then that's totally fine too. Go back to work if it helps to distract you. Just don't overload yourself – avoid working long hours and stay away from any stress!

Stick to your daily mindset routine. At the start of the month, you were filled with the hope and excitement of a new round of treatment, but now as you head into the 2WW, you may start to slip into feelings of doubt and anxiety as you go through the familiar agonizing wait. This is the *critical* time to keep going with your mindset routine – practise gratitude daily, repeat your positive affirmations and focus on your vision as much as possible. Really feel what it will be like to be a mum and allow yourself to get excited about those images. Use as many visual prompts as you can to bring your vision to life. Just go for it… you have absolutely nothing to lose and everything to gain.

Self-care is your priority. What can you do over the next two weeks to look after yourself? What makes you happy? You are the absolute priority in these two weeks, so it's imperative that you create time for yourself to do the small things you enjoy. It could be simple things: having a relaxing soak in the bath, connecting with nature by going for a walk, going to the cinema or going out for dinner. You could also book an outing for you and your partner, or your friends and family. Focus on things that make you feel happy and indulge yourself by filling those two weeks with activities that are all about you.

Laughter is the best medicine. Anything that makes you laugh is great for your mindset too. The benefits are endless. Laughing keeps you present and stops you worrying about whether or not you might be pregnant. It relaxes you and releases endorphins. In short, it simply makes you feel happier. Arrange a movie night for you and your partner to watch your favourite comedy, or follow your favourite comedian online and watch a clip every night before you go to sleep.

Create a visible plan for the 2WW. Work out your plan for how you will fill those 14 days in advance so that you know what you're doing. Stick it on the fridge or get it up on your phone. Fill those two weeks with activities that promote self-care, give you a positive mindset and make you happy, in whatever way works for you. For some people, this will mean keeping their mind busy by going back to work or booking some outings; for others, it could be having some lazy days at home. Build in mindset activities every day too and give yourself some treats! Create milestones at regular intervals during the two weeks so that you have little things to look forward to. Be creative with your plan and make it fun. Having a plan to follow will give a positive structure to the two weeks and keep you distracted.

A shorter 2WW. And finally, there is some good news if you are on the 2WW for fertility treatment. Due to medical advances, the two-week wait is reducing – hurrah! Depending on what treatment you are following and the particular process in your clinic, you may be offered a blood test to see if you are pregnant part way through the two-week wait. This could be as early as day eight after ovulation, so the wait may be a lot shorter. But every clinic is very different, so do make sure you talk this through with your consultant beforehand so you are fully aware of the process you will be going through, and ultimately how long you will have to wait!

CHAPTER 28

HAVING A BABY IN YOUR 40s

This is one I know all about. In Chapter 9, I spoke about how turning 40 is an invisible deadline for those who are trying to conceive. For some reason, we all want to be pregnant before this milestone age. This could be due, in some part, to the well-documented medical risks associated with having a baby once you turn 40. Or it could be due to society's view of being a new mum in your 40s. Babies are hard work, and we all want the energy to cope with the sleepless nights and toddlers tearing around the house. We don't want to be the old mum in the playground and, of course, we want to be around for as much of our children's lives as possible.

For whatever reason, things don't always work out according to the timeline we had in our heads when we were younger. Many people, including me, go on to have children in their 40s. So, what are the benefits of being a Mum when you are the wrong side of 40?

Maturity. In your 40s you have a lot more life experience under your belt than a mum in their 20s or 30s, which is likely to mean you are more emotionally mature. Looking back, my 20s and 30s were all about me! By the time I reached 40, I was lot less selfish and much more patient, which meant I felt "ready" to look after another human being 24/7 and I was happy to miss out on all the parties and social gatherings, as I'd got those out of my system already. Life took on a new phase and I was ready to embrace it.

With that maturity comes more self-discipline, which I believe rubs off on your children. I was definitely more structured and disciplined with my approach to parenting than I would have been when I was younger. I'm not saying that is necessarily the right way to do things (everyone is different, after all!), but for me it worked really well, and it has instilled some good habits in the children which I've noticed as they are growing up. Although, let's remember that I did have triplets, so a degree of structure and organization was critical for survival!

Financial security. My first pregnancy was 20 years after my school friend's first pregnancy. She was 21 when she had her first child, and I was 41! Having children so much later in life meant that I was working for a lot longer before I finally went on maternity leave. My husband and I were both working full time during those extra 20 years, which meant that once the children finally came along, we had already built up our careers, we'd had a mortgage for a number of years and we were in a better position financially than when we had started out. I was more established in my job when I finally got pregnant and had some solid experience under my belt. This meant there was less risk of my career falling behind if I took some time off, which can be a worry for younger mums with potentially only a few years' work experience behind them.

As the children have got older, we have come to realize that they are very expensive! They may have nursery costs when they are babies and toddlers, and then there are all the nappies! They are constantly growing, which means they always need new clothes (hand-me-downs are a life saver), and once they start school, all the activities begin. And let's not forget Christmas and birthdays – and the family holidays! It has helped enormously to have more financial security behind us, and it takes the pressure off both of us having to go back to high-pressure, high-earning roles. I have been able to choose a job with more flexibility, which works well for us.

Wisdom from friends. Another benefit of being an older mum is that your friends with older children hold the key to many pearls of wisdom when it comes to parenting. They have been there, done that, and they have definitely got the T-shirt – often two or three times over. They know exactly what to expect at every stage, they have made their mistakes and learnt from them, and they are very happy to pass on these invaluable nuggets of wisdom to you as the newbie.

They also have wardrobes and drawers full of hand-me-down clothes and toys that they will be more than happy for you to take off their hands. Another bonus!

Downsides

In the spirit of objectivity, and being totally honest, I'm not going to lie to you… there are a few downsides of being an older mum. I'm mentioning them to be transparent and because it's good to go into these things with your eyes wide open. Yes, it is more tiring when you're older. Kids are full-on and, particularly when they are babies, the lack of sleep on top of being older can be hard to cope with. Children require a lot of energy, from all the practical things you need to do during the day to look after them, to all the night feeds and interrupted sleep. And then, once they are toddling about, they have boundless energy and require a lot of entertaining. Be prepared to be on your knees building train tracks or playing with Barbies one minute and then chasing them around the local park the next, without a chance to sit down for a cup of tea in between.

If I'm honest, this wasn't a problem for me in my early 40s – I actually felt in my prime back then. I have noticed it more recently though, since being over 45. Everyone has their own energy levels and, to be honest, having a baby is so all-consuming in the beginning that I defy the most energetic of people not to feel tired. You will feel exhausted while you adjust to the new routine and get used to being woken up regularly in the night. But it is very unlikely you will be disappointed you haven't got the energy to go on a big night out because

I'm pretty confident that you won't want one, whatever age you may be! (But it's still important to book these in from time to time.)

Ten years on, yes, I might be one of the older mums in the playground, but I've got over that now too. When I look at my NCT group that I first met when we were all pregnant and I was 40, we were such an eclectic group of different personalities, nationalities and ages. But we all got on famously because of our experience of being pregnant together and our shared connection from having our babies. That meant that age didn't matter. We built such a strong bond during that first year and we supported each other in such a unique and special way (and, by the way, joining NCT or another baby group is a must for invaluable support when you do have your baby).

Having said that, there can be observations and preconceptions from people around you when you are out and about. A dear friend of mine who had her second child at 47 told me that she often got comments from people she met during her day. She had more than a few shocking tales to tell, including a woman at her toddler group who turned to her child and said, "Aah, are you out with your granny today?" That wouldn't have been great for her confidence on the best of days, but it was especially bad when she was exhausted after no sleep, but she had managed to make the effort to shower and put some make-up on! Isn't it incredible what people come out with?!

But really, these downsides are trivial compared to the benefits. Having a baby is a wonderful experience that will bring you so much joy, love and laughter that I can only begin to describe. Whatever age you embark on this adventure, there will be benefits and downsides. So, if you are worried about being an older mum, the most important thing for you to do is to push aside the premeditated timeline that has been lurking inside your head. Look back at Chapter 8 to help you work through this and keep reminding yourself that you are having your baby at exactly the right time for YOU.

CHAPTER 29

TAKING A BREAK FROM TRYING TO CONCEIVE

If you reach a point where trying to conceive is dominating your life and taking its toll on you both emotionally and physically, it could be time to take a break. It may even be time to stop for good.

The latter may be hard to imagine. I know from my own experience that it is hugely difficult to make the decision to stop completely and draw a line under your dreams of getting pregnant. When we had reached our breaking point, I decided to take a three-month break. I have always believed that making decisions in life when you are stressed, upset or angry never ends well. For me, I wanted to see how I felt after a short break rather than making such a big decision when I was so stressed and physically exhausted from it all. So, what are the signs that you should take a break, or even stop trying completely?

- You are exhausted, mentally and physically, and you have the lost the joy in life.
- You become obsessed with getting pregnant naturally and refuse to admit there may be a medical issue.
- You are avoiding seeing a doctor or specialist to investigate your fertility.
- Your struggle is affecting your relationships – you are losing your connection and communication is breaking down.

- You are struggling to cope with your job on top of your fertility journey.
- Your friendships are breaking down as you are isolating yourself, avoiding going out and withdrawing from social situations.
- Your mental health is on the edge, and you feel unable to talk to anyone about it.
- You have no idea where to go next with your quest to conceive.

If some or all of these phrases describe you, it may be time to pause or stop trying to conceive. Here's how to make the transition easy:

Make it a clean break. If you're going to have a break from trying to conceive, make it a clean break. Put away the ovulation kits and fertility apps and do your very best to stop monitoring your monthly cycle for a few months. Have sex when you want to instead of at the right time of the month. Avoid analysing your body at every stage of the month. I remember finding this particularly hard at first – after all, you want to give your body every chance. But remind yourself why you're doing this. The break is only a few months, and your body will be better off for the physical break and lower stress levels.

Stop reading pregnancy books and articles, stop listening to the podcasts and come off any fertility sites. Believe me, this will be so refreshing! Fill your time with more leisurely and relaxing activities instead. Find a different kind of podcast on a completely new subject or read a fiction book that has been on your list for a while.

Get back to the fun stuff in life. If you're like me, you will have put your life on hold while trying to conceive. I can remember saying that I didn't want to book a holiday or train for a running challenge just in case I was pregnant. Now is the time to cast all those fears aside! When I decided to take my break, we had recently moved house and the garden was a total mess. It was Easter and I threw myself into the gardening project. It was the perfect distraction and a good way of practising mindfulness. Think about what YOU have been putting off in life. Book that amazing holiday you have been too scared to commit to or sign up for that 10k run (or even a marathon!). Take your life off the pause button as much as possible and do what makes you happy – whether it's social events, house renovations, day trips or weekends away.

CHAPTER 30

DECIDING TO STOP FOR GOOD

It takes a lot of courage to stop trying for good, and it's not an overnight decision. If you are faced with a bereavement in life, you know it is final as the person is never coming back. Over time, you can begin to process their loss and start to move on with your life. But when you stop trying for a baby, nothing is ever certain. There is no end to the underlying hope that something may change in the future. Even though you are not officially trying, you may still pray for a little miracle each month and catch yourself dreaming of a different life. This means that it takes a lot longer to accept the loss of not having a baby that could still possibly arrive.

Chances are you will know when the time is right to stop trying. A bit like when you are taking a break, you will know when you have fully exhausted all the medical options and you are physically and emotionally spent. Your life has been on pause for months, often years, and deep down you know the time has come for this to change.

Once you have made the decision, you may feel nervous about sharing it with your partner. Will they feel the same way? What happens if they don't want to stop? You can't know how they are feeling until you talk to them, but sometimes the response you get is relief. After all, they just want what's best for you, and you may find that they even admit they were only going along with it to keep you happy.

Give yourself time. Once you are both on the same page, give yourself time to come to terms with such a big decision and allow yourself to go through all the emotions that will inevitably follow. You are not going to process this one overnight. Keep talking to your partner and share how you're both feeling. Be ready to experience a whole host of emotions. You may feel sad about your decision at first and experience an outpouring of grief or loss. Or you may feel numb for a while and then be hit with a wave of emotions later on.

Process your emotions. When these emotions do hit, the worst thing you can do is suppress them or pretend they're not happening. Talking to your partner is key, of course – chances are they are feeling something similar. Counselling can be a valuable outlet to help you process both your decision and all the emotions that come with it, whether you feel grief, loss, sadness or depression. These emotions can take hold if not properly released, which can result in physical illness. When I was 30, my father died, and I had a terrible eczema patch develop on my hand. It was there for months. A few years later, when I was researching Chinese medicine as an alternative therapy for pregnancy, I discovered the Five Element theory, and the metal element's link to the emotion of grief (look it up, it's really interesting how emotions affect the body physically). Eczema and other skin conditions can often appear when the metal element is unbalanced, and looking back, I didn't really talk about how I felt after my Dad died; I just buried it all and got on with my busy life. But the emotions were still there, and they manifested themselves physically.

Consult your community. If you don't have the right people around you to talk to, consider going back to your fertility community. Chances are there are many women facing the exact same decision you are, and this provides a safe space for you to open up about your feelings. This community knows better than anyone what it's like to be battling this decision, and can offer comforting words and share their own personal insights to help you with yours.

Tell people. There comes a point when you will want to share your decision with your close circle. You may wait a while until you reach a point when you can talk about the situation without getting upset. Once you take this step, be prepared for some mixed reactions! Some people will be happy for you and support your decision. After all, they just want what's best for you. But the others! The need to say the right thing or make you hang on to hope even longer can be overwhelming for some. Out will come those well-meaning comments again, such as, "Maybe now you're not trying it will happen," or, "Well, it could still happen, especially now you're relaxed!"

These comments are said with the best intentions but without any understanding of the enormity of your decision and the heartbreaking journey that you have gone through to get to this point. Internally you'll be screaming, "Did you not hear me? We have stopped trying!" Think about how you will handle these types of comments and what your response will be. You may find the easiest response is just to laugh it off while clenching your fists behind your back. Or you may want to be more direct and remind them that you have actually stopped for good, and it would be nice to have their support.

Make a new plan for life. When we did our fifth IVF, we knew it would be our last. We knew that if we finally decided to stop trying, we needed to create an alternative dream. For us this was going to be buying a holiday home abroad. In the end, we never got to that stage, but nevertheless, it was something that we were excited about.

Once you make the decision to stop trying, there is a gaping hole in your life, not only from the loss of having the baby you dreamed about, but from all the time and effort in trying to get pregnant. Now you need a new dream to fill this hole, something you can both throw yourself into that will bring you some long-awaited joy. Sit down with your partner and make a plan. What is your new project going to be? The options are endless! It could be getting a pet, moving house, moving to another country, starting a new business, learning a new skill or changing your life in some other way. No, you don't have the baby, but what you do have is the time and the possibility to achieve something else fulfilling in life. It doesn't have to be enormous; it can just be something simple you do to refocus on an alternative future together.

CHAPTER 31

CONSIDERING A DIFFERENT PATH TO A FAMILY

These days there are many different ways to create a family. If you have exhausted all the medical procedures for having your own baby and you still haven't been successful, you may want to consider other options, such as donor eggs, donor sperm, surrogacy or adoption. It may be hard to accept one of these routes at first and give up on your dream of having a baby that you created, but try and look at this from a different perspective. The child you have this way is still your own child in every other sense, and in many cases, you will be the only parent they will ever know.

The internet is filled with inspirational stories of adoption and surrogacy, and the list of celebrities going down this route is endless. Often, your chances of success are higher if you go down one of these routes rather than trying naturally or via the more traditional avenues. For example, if you are over 40 with low egg quality and are considering using a donor egg, you know that the donor eggs are of the highest quality and come from a young, healthy female at the peak of her fertility. Ask your consultant about the success rates for donors and compare this to the averages for your own age. And do look into the rules regarding donor anonymity as these are evolving over time, and therefore should be a consideration too.

Having said all this, starting a family via any of these routes is still complex. Adoption and surrogacy can be expensive and time-consuming. These days there aren't as many babies available for adoption in the UK, which is why people often go overseas. This can be both expensive and unreliable. Of course, the celebrities make it look easy, but very often we don't see all the time and effort spent behind the scenes before they produce their happy ending on the front page of *Hello magazine*. Adopting an older child in the UK can be cheaper than going overseas, but there are still complex assessment processes and criteria in place. And there are other things to consider with adopting an older child. Parents may be concerned about the emotional baggage that might come with the child and the fact that they have missed out on their early life. However, there are many wonderful success stories out there and many benefits of adopting an older child. An older child can articulate their feelings and experiences as you go through the process together, and of course there are still plenty more big "firsts" to be there for in their life.

The best thing you can do when considering any of these options is research, research, research. Find out as much as you can about the different routes available to you. Speak to people who have gone down that route and been successful. Ask medical professionals for their advice. Join an online community for the option you're interested in exploring. When you only have limited information to hand, you are more likely to shut down a new idea prematurely without giving it due consideration. Or you might be scared off by the complexity of it all. Keep an open mind and make an informed decision when you have the objective facts in front of you, coupled with a number of different perspectives. As I have spoken about in this book, thinking positively is key to being open to new possibilities as they arise and will avoid you dismissing an idea before it's even started.

FINAL THOUGHTS

Thank you for sticking with me on this journey of discovery. You have come a long way since you started this book – well done! No doubt there has been a lot of self-reflection, which may have been painful at times. I'm hoping that you have come to realize that you are not alone on this very tough journey, even though it may feel like it. I hope you are reassured that you are not the only one who is completely overwhelmed and has regular mindset meltdowns. I also hope that you are now taking back control of your mindset by putting into practice the tools I have shared and working out your own personal action plan to move you forward.

So many people read a self-help book and then don't do anything with it. Remember one of my favourite quotes – nothing changes when nothing changes! If you have started to put into practice the tools in this book, then you should be super proud of yourself! You have made a big investment in yourself mentally and that is definitely a trophy moment that you should congratulate yourself for! I'm also hoping that my survival guides can be a reference point for you as you continue through this journey, and a reminder to put your own self-care at the top of your priority list. Be compassionate with yourself and be your own biggest supporter. That means doing everything you can to look after yourself and put yourself first.

Be fully committed

My final thought is something that underpins all of the work you have done in this book. The last thing I ask of you is to approach your fertility journey by being fully committed. Give it absolutely everything you have got. Let me give you an example. If you are going into IVF, you are investing so much in the process. Financially, you are spending a shedload of money. Physically, you are putting your body through so much. Time-wise, you are juggling appointments with a busy job and finding the time to attend last-minute blood tests and scans at the drop of a hat.

But what about your mental investment? Are you giving it everything mentally too? Are you walking into the next stage of your fertility journey with a positive attitude and an open mind – a bit like a boxer walking out to the ring, fired up, energetic and ready for anything? Or do you allow your mind to fill with worries, doubts and anxiety? Are you holding on to the disappointments of the past? Even the tiniest voice of doubt in your head has an impact on your thinking.

If that's the case, I want to remind you that you have the power to change those thoughts. Make a commitment to yourself to be fully invested mentally as well as every other way. You have invested so much – you do not want to be the one letting yourself down by having a mindset meltdown. Treat this goal of getting pregnant like any other big project in your life. Be fully committed to it, believe in it, and create a mindset that goes out and makes it happen! Be open and positive about the future. Yes, there will be ups and downs, moments of hope and days of disappointment. But the tools you have learnt can help you recover, bounce back quickly and get you back on track.

Toward the end of my journey, I felt out of control, anxious and terrified about a future without children. I didn't realize I was the one creating this reality in my head. I was at my lowest point back then. Chances are, you have read this book because you were at your lowest point too. You had no idea what to do next and you believed you had tried everything.

Now you are in a different place. You are fully equipped with the tools to change what's going on in your head and you can start this right NOW! By being fully committed and practising these tools daily, you will create new patterns of thinking and you will see your feelings and behaviours change for the better. This will get your fertility plan back on track, and I assure you that life will feel better.

These tools are a gift, not just for your fertility journey, but for life. I have used them many times as I have embarked on the challenges of parenting, and they have helped me since then with managing triplets as they grow up, as well as my other life projects. They always help me bounce back, find new strategies and move forward in life. I pray you will get the same benefit and find your happy ending, whatever that looks like. You so deserve it.

ACKNOWLEDGEMENTS

I first started thinking about writing this book when the triplets were tiny. When I was doing the endless night feeds, I would gaze at my three little miracles in total wonder of what I had finally produced. Thank you to Jessica, Harry and Max for being the most perfect reward after such a long and very tough journey. You are the light of my life, and you bring so much joy into our world every day. Right from the start, your fun-loving, happy personalities have shone through, and I am so proud of each of you in every way. You are one hundred percent my inspiration for this book.

To Rob… I couldn't have been on this journey with a better person. Thanks for supporting me with this project from the start. You listened to my crazy ideas and gave me all the support I needed without question. And thank you for being my absolute rock on our fertility journey – I always felt so loved and supported. Even though it was the toughest time, it gave us the opportunity to have some amazing experiences together, just us, which I appreciate so much more now looking back (note to those trying to get pregnant – do lots together while you still can!). And once those babies arrived, you were the best triplet dad there could be. We embraced the chaos together and we were a fantastic team. Thank you xxx

Thanks to my incredible family, who have always supported me in everything I do. Mum and Jim for being there for me… ALWAYS. Rob and I could not have survived the triplet baby days without your selfless support, and the children have always adored you. What special memories we have with you both – that holiday in Crete, wow! And Mum, you are still so hands-on and we love you for it. Jane, my sister, my rock and my biggest supporter in every way: I literally could not get through life without you, and there is so much more to thank you for than just this book! Your loyalty, friendship and unwavering support in everything I do is one of the most special things in my life. As we always say, we are so lucky to have each other, and we are carbon copies now more than ever!

A big thank you to my Uncle David for your personal support on this project, it is truly appreciated. Louise – my second sister and parenting mentor – I love you loads! And my very special in-laws, Vicky and John, thank you for juggling your much-valued grandparent support with a house-renovation project when the kids were babies and, of course, for paying for our final round of IVF. Who would have known what value for money you would get – three for the price of one! Thanks to **all** my extended family for supporting the book from the start – the Cooks, Sears, Baileys, Everndens, Williamsons and of course our fabulous Allder nephews.

A special mention to my school friends – the Mag 7. What can I say… a 40-year friendship that I am grateful for every day. Rach, your endless enthusiasm for the book and positive contributions have been so appreciated throughout. And Holly has come into her own with the book cover input – thank you so much! Claire, thank you for letting me play mum with Jeanie and Rosie when I couldn't have my own – I'll treasure those memories. Linner, thank you for being a huge support to me when I was trying to get pregnant, and for always taking my desperate phone calls, even when you were juggling three small kids of your own! Ing, thank you for always being so considerate of me when you told me about your pregnancies, I'll never forget the concerned look on your face when you told me about Josh! And thank you ladies for my five Mag 7 godchildren – Rachael, Jeanie, Rosie, Arthur and Daisy. Most of them are grown up now, but they were the perfect distraction for me when I couldn't have my own – I loved every minute of that time, and I had a lot more energy back then too!

Becca, my infertility soulmate. Looking back, we were so lucky to navigate the ups and downs of our fertility journey together. I couldn't have got through it without you. Thank you for laughing with me and crying with me; for all the daily "on the way to work calls"; for listening patiently to my latest mindset techniques; for being my IVF buddy, and for generally being the person who "gets it", mainly because you were going through exactly the same experience as me. We are eternally grateful to the universe for producing Daisy only three months after mine came along. Ask, Believe, Receive ☺

Special thanks go to Roz Wilson-Carr, member of the Mag 7 and my personal proofreader for this book project. Thanks for your expertise, invaluable insights and endless patience. Your calm response when at the last minute I said, "Can you do this by tomorrow?!" was always appreciated, and I am so grateful for all your proof-reading talents and valuable feedback, right from the start. Thanks also to Ian Moore (an old friend and now a *Sunday Times* bestselling author), for mentoring me at the start of the publishing process and encouraging me to aim high. It certainly paid off. A huge thank you goes to Wendy Yorke, my wonderful book agent, who I found just at the right time. Thank you for taking a chance on my book and believing in it – our manifesting worked! Thanks also to Emma Lord for first introducing me to Rhonda and *The Secret* back in 2005, the book that changed everything for me. And a special mention to my dear friend Julie, who has been a constant in our parallel lives for over 30 years… a kindred spirit who inspires me more than she knows.

To all my mum friends – who would have thought that having children could bring the most wonderful new friends into your life who would then champion this book project from the start? Thank you to all you lovely ladies – school mums, neighbours and my wonderful NCT group. Special mention to my local crew who have been so supportive, especially when I was doubting myself at the start. Vicky, for all your positive interest in the book and for always boosting my confidence. Jo for the invaluable (and very positive!) feedback from someone who has been there and gets it, and of course Natalie – my multiples partner in crime. From that first outing to Wisley, we have created the most special memories with those five babies and the added bonus of a little godson later. Rob and I couldn't have got through the early triplet chaos without the support and friendship of you and Jim – we love you loads!

I talk about acupuncture in this book, and I wanted to give a special mention to the best kept secret in Guildford – Wendy Wang, the most wonderful acupuncturist who is a hormone specialist and is now helping me navigate the challenges of menopause – eek! Her acupuncture is like no other, the most calming and relaxing experience ever. I recommended two people to Wendy who both fell pregnant within a month of seeing her, so if you're local, do check her out – she sees clients at Neal's Yard in Guildford. Wendy is a hidden gem who I wish I'd had the pleasure of knowing when I was on my journey.

Thank you to my previous clients who have given me the most wonderful reviews for this book. And not forgetting Koja Coffee in Guildford. Thank you for having the most delicious black tea (in a pot, of course) and the best carrot cake I have ever had. You kept me well fuelled for the many hours of writing, and I was totally gutted when you moved!

And finally, to my Dad. Sadly, he's not been with us for a long time, but he's never been forgotten. I know he would have loved his triplet grandchildren, especially having two boys that love sport almost as much as he did in a house full of girls! Thank you for giving me the drive, resilience and resourcefulness to succeed in life. I don't think I fully appreciated those gifts until now.

RECOMMENDED READING – SOME BOOKS THAT HAVE INSPIRED ME ON THIS JOURNEY

The Secret – Rhonda Byrne

The Power – Rhonda Byrne

You Can Heal Your Life – Louise Hay

Solve for Happy – Mo Gawdat

Breaking the Habits of Being Yourself – Jo Dispenza

The Choice – Edith Eger

The Power of Now – Eckhart Tolle

The Power of Meditation – Sharon Salzberg

10% Happier – Dan Harris

Overcoming Anxiety – Gill Hasson

The Happiness Advantage – Shawn Achor

A Little Light on the Spiritual Laws – Diana Cooper

Thoughts are Things – Bob Proctor and Greg S. Reid

Happy Mind, Happy Life – Dr Rangan Chatterjee

Stop Thinking Start Living – Richard Carlson

Your Mind Can Heal Your Body – Matthew Manning

The Secrets of Meditation – Davidji

ABOUT CHERISH EDITIONS

Cherish Editions is a bespoke publishing service for authors of mental health, wellbeing and inspirational books.

As a division of Trigger Publishing, the UK's leading independent mental health and wellbeing publisher, we are experienced in creating and selling positive, responsible, important and inspirational books, which work to de-stigmatize the issues around mental health and improve the mental health and wellbeing of those who read our titles.

Founded by Adam Shaw, a mental health advocate, author and philanthropist, and leading psychologist Lauren Callaghan, Cherish Editions aims to publish books that provide advice, support and inspiration. We nurture our authors so that their stories can unfurl on the page, helping them to share their uplifting and moving stories.

Cherish Editions is unique in that a percentage of the profits from the sale of our books goes directly to leading mental health charity Shawmind, to deliver its vision to provide support for those experiencing mental ill health.

Find out more about Cherish Editions by visiting cherisheditions.com or joining us on:
Twitter @cherisheditions
Facebook @cherisheditions
Instagram @cherisheditions

Cherish
EDITIONS

ABOUT SHAWMIND

A proportion of profits from the sale of all Trigger books go to their sister charity, Shawmind, also founded by Adam Shaw and Lauren Callaghan. The charity aims to ensure that everyone has access to mental health resources whenever they need them.

Find out more about the work Shawmind do by visiting shawmind.org or joining them on:
Twitter @Shawmind_
Facebook @ShawmindUK
Instagram @Shawmind_

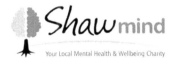

Milton Keynes UK
Ingram Content Group UK Ltd.
UKHW020946241023
431236UK00006B/51

9 781915 680655